Annabel Smoker

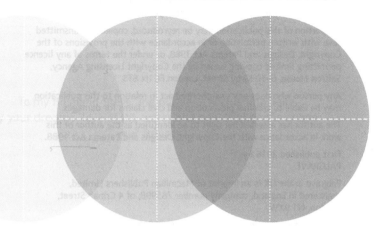

# Launching Your Career in Nursing and Midwifery

## A Practical Guide

macmillan education    palgrave

# Foreword

Graduating and starting your first post as a newly qualified nurse or midwife is a huge moment of transition. From the relatively protected world of university where choices are largely made for you to starting in the world of work, either for the first time or anew following university, is both exciting and stressful. An array of choices and opportunities seem to be set out in front of you but there is also great pressure to "get onto the career ladder" and secure your first post amidst all your peers who seem to be racing to achieve the same goal.

While graduating nurses and midwives are much sought after, securing the right first job is an important one as it provides a platform for all that follows, both in early career experience and also in the opportunities it affords for hopefully a long, rich and stimulating career ahead. It is however worth remembering that this is a two-way process. Your prospective employer is seeking to choose an individual who they believe will be the best fit for their organisation and has the attributes and competencies they require. You, on the other hand, are seeking an employer who will support you as an individual and your future career and an organisation that is committed to you. Make sure you focus on the latter as much as on demonstrating what you have to offer. The first months and years after graduating are known to be stressful and demanding and sustaining yourself through these while putting the building blocks of professional experience in place is difficult. An employer that pays great attention to how you are supported through this and who offers ongoing training opportunities could be what makes your next step successful or not. These are questions for you to ask of prospective employers.

This book is a wonderful resource for all on the brink of this journey. It is practical and also full of tips and techniques for making crucial choices and succeeding through the hoops of employment selection processes. Remember, though, that this is not the end of the story but the beginning of a career journey which if anything like my own is invisible at this point, but full of opportunity. Seize the moment and enjoy what lies ahead.

Professor Dame Jessica Corner
Dean of Faculty of Health Sciences, University of Southampton

Currently there is no national data about the number of nurses employed outside of the NHS, but market intelligence shows this is where opportunities have increased significantly over the past 10 years. As a result of the politically influenced model of the contracting of professional healthcare services, both within and without the NHS, future nurse employment will inevitably follow different pathways than the well-established "NHS Band 5" newly qualified role. In order to understand how the healthcare landscape might look in the future and where new opportunities will be, it is worth reading the executive summaries of two key documents, the NHS Five Year Forward View (NHS England 2014) and the Dalton Review (DH 2014b).

## WHO CAN HELP ME?

Career advice and counselling has its place at every turning point in your career. It can take various forms, from informal, unsolicited information given by a supportive mentor or clinical manager to discussions at one-to-one progress reviews with your tutor, within employability themed modules, or comprise formally arranged sessions with a designated careers counsellor/advisors/practitioner. The term "counselling" (Oxford English Dictionary 2015) means the provision of professional assistance and guidance in resolving personal or psychological problems. You may reasonably feel the term "problems" has negative connotations, so perhaps thinking about resolving "dilemmas" or "challenges" is more helpful. However, turning to a careers counsellor to find direction is not necessarily everyone's first response to a dilemma or challenging time.

Experience indicates that some students will seek expert help only after an adverse event, such as following an interview where they were unsuccessful in gaining employment. The reason often is that they felt they could manage themselves and did not like to ask for help. At the other end of the spectrum are students who, with good reason, start the process well before their final year: they exploit every step of the career planning cycle (Chapter 2), all available avenues of support, checking and cross-checking information with military precision prior to making any key decision.

Accessing help is not perceived as a weakness by those whose role is to guide students through what is a testing process; indeed contributing to a person's successful achievement of their dream job is very satisfying. Employability is high on every university agenda, and this theme is frequently an established thread in programmes from year one to graduation. Arguably, instead of being a discrete activity that occurs mainly in the final year, timely career guidance should be overt from the point of your undergraduate application in the recruitment process and should be available to all students throughout their programmes. So if you are reading this and are now worried that you do not know whom to contact in your institution, then it is time to identify who can help you.

In addition to specialist employability leads within faculties, there are often career practitioners or coaches employed by university careers services who are aligned to a faculty or programme. These staff have discipline-specific knowledge and provide bespoke advice and support at every stage from pre-employment to beyond. For a defined period of time after completion many universities offer their alumni continued access to expert help when, for example, an individual is contemplating a subsequent job move, return to study or career change. This support may be in the form of face-to-face meetings or increasingly, with tech-nological developments, online via email or Skype.

Furthermore the prospective employer is a key resource. You will have already built up a network of clinical contacts, and this will be invaluable. How to exploit this will be examined in more detail in Chapter 2, section "Step 2: Exploring options". Utilising both your university and contacts early is advisable. Looking after your own interests and making sure you are as prepared as possible can prevent avoidable mistakes.

## CAREER PLANNING THEORIES

There are a number of different ways to approach the career decision-making process; an awareness of some career theory can help you understand how your career decisions might be influenced and shift over time as your priorities naturally change. Four of the main career development theories are summarised in Table 1.2. The Structural or Opportunity Structure theory (Roberts 1968) argues that career choice does not rest solely with you (the applicant) and that your decisions are controlled by the interplay of environmental factors outside of your control, such as the offer of a university place and the availability of jobs when you graduate. Add to this sociocultural aspects such as gender, class background, ethnicity or disability and self-imposed constraints which may limit your horizon. For example, some choices you make may be influenced by what you value, or believe others to value rather than what would be the most satisfying for you personally. The environment and a person's upbringing can restrict the options they explore, ruling themselves out of certain roles and what they might aspire to achieve. If

**TABLE 1.2  Different career planning theories**

| Structural or Opportunity Structure theory | Person-Environment Fit theory |
|---|---|
| • It is important to be aware of the job market and what is on offer.<br>• You do not have sole control over your future career; the economy and employers play a significant part too.<br>• Not securing a job can be down to issues with the economy, not just your suitability.<br>• Job status is important to you/others.<br>• There may be opportunities that you overlook. | • Categorises personality types and work environments.<br>• Identifies occupations/environments which match your individual characteristics.<br>• Develops good self-awareness of the person you are and the person you may want to become in terms of your skills, motivations, interests and personal attributes. |
| **Developmental theory** | **Planned Happenstance theory** |
| • Good career decisions involve taking short and longer term views.<br>• It is a continuous process, so you need to revisit decisions on a regular basis.<br>• This approach encourages you to experiment with different jobs before finding the right "fit" for you.<br>• What might be the right fit now may change significantly during your working life. | • The aim is to transform unplanned events into career opportunities.<br>• It is not always necessary to plan a career in the conventional sense.<br>• Instead it is important to prepare for happenstance (the unexpected).<br>• Focus on developing skills and attributes that could be useful in all sorts of situations.<br>• Be curious (find out about things related to work) and see chance events as opportunities that could lead to action. |

those around you, whose opinion/s you respect, do not support a choice this may discourage you from applying for certain jobs. Conversely, an environment with plenty of opportunities and solid networks can encourage people to be more ambitious and facilitate career development. An advantage of structural theories is that they can help put situations into perspective. The lack of opportunity or success is not wholly the applicant's fault because they cannot control some of the wider factors.

A different approach is the Person-Environment Fit theory (Holland 1997) which uses tools to categorise personality types and work environments to identify "best fit". Having this insight helps people choose environments to work in that are suited to their individual traits and preferences. The role of personality assessments will be examined in greater depth in Chapter 2.

Another perspective, the Developmental theory (Super 1957), sees career planning as a continuous process and reassures those who may be anxious of making a mistake that it is acceptable to experiment until they find what is right for them. What feels the right option now will almost certainly change with age, experience and new priorities, such as the need for a greater work–life balance and this opens up the notion of a second career.

The final theory offered here for consideration is that of Planned Happenstance (Mitchell et al 1999). Preparing graduates to take advantage of the unexpected or "serendipity" is important. The labour market fluctuates; when there are plenty of jobs applicants are in a stronger position and can move between employers with relative ease and security, knowing that if they subsequently find it is not the right job, then there are other options. However, when there is a shortage of jobs in particular areas, people can feel trapped by the lack of prospect. Having the courage to make a move and being in the right place at the right time are issues that are explored in more depth later.

Think about a theory or a blend of theories you prefer and why this is the case. Different elements of these theories feed into the career planning cycle, which is explored in Chapter 2.

- What are your interests?
- What aspects of work (work values) give you the greatest job satisfaction?
- Can you outline your strengths and areas for development?
- Do you know how you learn best?

Whilst some students will have a very clear idea about where they do and do not want to work, it is recognised that many struggle with making life-changing decisions and naturally worry about making mistakes. There are also those who have loved every placement to date and therefore find it difficult to choose. This is normal. Final year students who are making these decisions talk about knowing when it is the right choice because "It simply feels right", "I felt 100 per cent at home and part of the team", "I've found my niche" or "It was a place-ment I didn't want to leave". Conversely, exposure to an area of practice, before deciding whether or not to apply, may change a person's mind and this is important too. Instincts and intuition matter. The realisation that "I don't see myself here" and the relief that "I was glad to have this experience because it was not what I expected and this is actually not the place for me so I will cross it off the list of possibilities" stop people from making the wrong application.

Being honest with yourself and others is essential; if you feel uncomfortable, vulnerable, fearful or physically unwell in certain roles, then knowingly placing yourself in a position where you will not be properly supported or safe could be disastrous. For example, not eve-ryone copes with or is able to work night shifts and this may rule out those areas that expect staff to rotate onto nights. Others may prefer and thrive in a busy hospital ward environment as opposed to that of a community service where practitioners need to be more self-reliant, carry their own caseload and work independently in clients' homes. Of course, choices can be restricted if the 12-month period of preceptor-ship requires the NQ employee to rotate through a number of clinical areas, as in the case of some midwifery units where hospital and com-munity services are integrated and staff will be expected to be able to work all shifts.

Finances can also restrict choices if the role/location incurs addi-tional cost such as childcare, travel or parking. Short-term expedience may be the driving factor and the one which initially overrides the other less financially viable goals. Students may choose to move back home to reduce outgoings; with a regular income they can save for driving lessons and to buy a car which may be essential for a community post. The path to this goal should be thought through. This will help identify what will facilitate and what could potentially block progress towards this goal.

Myths regarding the level and type of experience required, for example, "you need to have worked on a hospital ward for 2 years before you can work in the community", are incredibly unhelpful, out of date and potentially undermine the confidence of a student, who would be well suited to apply for an NQ community role. It is therefore important to get sound advice, preferably from the recruiters themselves, to help inform your decision-making.

Many tools are available to support the early stages of career planning; however, few are specific to the needs of nursing and midwifery students. Undertaking the following reflective exercises (Activities 2.2 (Parts A and B) and 2.3) will help you to clarify and be more certain about the types of environment and clinical roles you like and ultimately where your real passion lies.

## ACTIVITY 2.2

### Part A "Tell the story"

Identify an (anonymised) situation from your student clinical practice where you were able to perform at your best. This may well be a relatively routine or repeated care practice rather than one that is memorable for its uniqueness; one "fragment" of a care episode will be sufficient. Make notes using the following headings:

1. What was the *situation*/context?
   - Who were the stakeholders?
   - What were the risks and to whom did they apply?
   - What legal/professional/care provider principles were applicable?
   - What constraints or challenges had to be addressed?

2. What *personal actions* did you undertake?
   - What decisions were you responsible for and what decisions did you make?
   - What theoretical/academic/research concepts did you consider?
   - What strategies did you subsequently use?
   - What was the result of your actions and how were the outcomes assessed?

### Part B Reflect on your "story"

In relation to the story above, now make notes under the following headings:
- What skills did you demonstrate in dealing with the situation?
- How does the situation described demonstrate your attitude to patients/clients?

- How would an independent observer in the situation describe your personal values?
- Why was the outcome rewarding for you?
- Is your own measurement of success different now compared to pre-university life?

If you have not, as part of this exercise, referred back to relevant excerpts from practice reports in your Assessment of Practice (AOP) or eFolio (electronic version of AOP) it may be worthwhile. There may be hard evidence, in the form of mentor comments, which substantiate your recollections; indeed these may also give extra detail.

The next activity, "How hungry am I?", is to help identify "how hungry" you are for a role or care setting by combining considerations of:

1. "Zeal and desires" – usually the things we enjoy the most or find most satisfying, and generally those that we are best at. This is suggestive of what we offer as a nurse or midwife.
2. "Personal strengths" – the ways we think, respond to and work with people and situations, often shaped by experiences of both life and caring. This tends to indicate how we will deliver our professional healthcare.
3. The two sets of data are then combined to identify your best offering to an employer that you will be able to deliver enjoyably. This may also identify gaps that can be addressed, for example, time or training.
4. Consider the time frame for your plans, that is, short, medium or longer term.

Table 2.1 provides an example compiled by a student, followed by an open-format table for you to complete (Activity 2.3).

| TABLE 2.1 "How hungry am I?" by Will, 27 (undergraduate mental health nurse) | |
|---|---|
| List your zeals and desires | 1. Nursing older adults with degenerative brain disorders<br>2. Taking responsibility for my own actions<br>3. Caring for clients over a prolonged period of time<br>4. Working independently<br>5. Working in clients' own homes with their families |
| List your personal strengths | 1. Listening to people more than talking to them<br>2. Learning about "old people" from my grandparents<br>3. My friend says I am more patient than he is<br>4. Strong families are the basis of strong communities<br>5. Older people have much to offer even if they are unwell |

**TABLE 2.1** *continued*

| | |
|---|---|
| Combine your lists of "zeals/desires" and "personal strengths" | 1. Community nursing of the elderly with mental ill health<br>2. Assessment of needs of client and their family to plan/ deliver long-term care, establishing these relationships<br>3. A specialist role, perhaps for Alzheimer's society or specialist NHS team<br>4. Cannot prescribe yet. Have additional pre-course experience as HCA |
| Identify your time frame/s (short, medium and long term) | 1. Initial NHS Band 5 job in hospital or community older adult mental health setting<br>2. Preceptorship. Practice as a RN<br>3. After 1 year apply for advanced clinical practice course and non-medical prescribing AND apply for Band 5 community jobs specific to degenerative brain disorders in older adults<br>4. Band 6 by 30th birthday |

**ACTIVITY 2.3**

### "How hungry am I?"

| | |
|---|---|
| List your zeals and desires | 1.<br>2.<br>3.<br>4.<br>5. |
| List your personal strengths | 1.<br>2.<br>3.<br>4.<br>5. |
| Combine your lists of "zeals/desires" and "personal strengths" | 1.<br>2.<br>3.<br>4.<br>5. |
| Identify your time frame/s (short, medium and long term) | 1.<br>2.<br>3.<br>4.<br>5. |

When looking at time frames you need to break these down into short-, medium- and long-term goals and be realistic. At this stage you may not know how long you might stay in a particular pay band before promotion, how quickly you can get onto courses, whether other qualifications are needed and how much experience, competence and confidence are required for a certain role, for example, to practise as an independent midwife or specialist nurse. In Chapter 6 former students reflect on their career pathways which give some insight into the preparatory steps necessary to secure more senior roles. These unanswered questions form your background research. In Step 2 when you are exploring options you will be able to fill in these gaps.

## PERSONALITY TYPE AND INFLUENCE ON CAREER CHOICES

At this early stage of planning for a career as a professional nurse or midwife it is useful to be forearmed with as much insight into yourself as possible. In addition to the preceding exercises understanding your own personality type is beneficial. The theories of Carl Jung (1971) remain amongst the most influential concepts, forming the basis of several personality-type assessments.

Graduating nurses and midwives may well have explored personality within their studies on psychological perspectives. However, informative personality assessment tools include:

- The Kiersey Temperament Sorter. This is a widely used personality instrument that helps people to identify their personality type. The tool is freely available via the Kiersey website: www.keirsey.com
- The Jung Typology Test is linked to research that generated the Myers-Briggs Type Indicator (1962 cited in the Myers-Briggs Foundation 2014). This tool is available free via the Human metrics website: www.humanmetrics.com

A further very simple but frequently highly accurate "tool" is to ask a close friend (but not a partner) "What sort of person am I really like?" Typically the first response will be both honest and insightful!

One could reasonably ask, "So what and why does personality matter if I can do the job?" Fundamentally, employing people with different backgrounds, cultures, talents and perspectives benefits both the workforce and the people it serves. New staff have to be able to work effectively with others as part of a team caring for people with individual needs. The recruiter will therefore be trying to image you as part of the team; conversely you will be thinking "Can I work with these people or in this environment?" Some organisations will use psychometric tests to screen candidates to ensure that they will "fit in"; even with practice it is very difficult to bluff answers in validated screening tools to project the type of persona that you think the recruiter is seeking. Furthermore if you have insight into how others see you and what the personality tests say about you then arguably you can constructively use this to your advantage.

## THE SWOT ANALYSIS

A SWOT analysis is a subjective assessment of information relating to the present and the future. It lends itself nicely to career planning as it facilitates pre-emptive thinking rather than encouraging a reliance on traditional reactions to circumstances. Data is structured logically to support and determine understanding, presentation, discussion and decision-making. The long-established tool is utilised in many settings, including business, marketing, manufacturing and more recently healthcare where it features in many AOP documents. As with many established tools there are many variants of SWOT yet the original core concept is applicable for career planning. In its simplest form, SWOT analysis remains as sequential consideration of Strengths, Weaknesses, Opportunities and Threats.

This can be simply undertaken in an individual reflection or as a group "brainstorm". Refer to Zoe's example in Box 2.1. Conceptualising strengths and weaknesses as internal and "in the present" factors and opportunities and threats as external and in the future factors can be more useful in immediate decision-making.

**BOX 2.1 Example SWOT analysis for Zoe, 21, midwifery graduate seeking Band 5 role in an NHS midwifery unit**

| STRENGTHS (internal) | WEAKNESSES (internal) |
| --- | --- |
| • I can easily demonstrate that I fulfil all the essential criteria. P5 grades were encouraging. <br> • Confidence has grown due to recent supervised caseload experience and involvement in parent education classes. <br> • My mentor appraisals support my ability to deal with high-risk births. <br> • I am not scared to ask for help. <br> • Hardworking, have high standards and am keen to learn. | • I get quite nervous which could affect my chance of success at interview. <br> • Timekeeping. I tend to leave things to the last minute but can't afford to miss NHS Jobs' deadline as won't secure an interview. <br> • The person specification asks for a current driving licence but I've not yet passed my test. |

| OPPORTUNITIES (external) | THREATS (external) |
|---|---|
| • To develop management skills in final placement with community midwives.<br>• Tutor and careers adviser both offering to review my applications and 1:1 mock interview practice.<br>• Band 5 pay – immediate assured income (in debt)!<br>• Multiple vacancies in local area, particularly in hospital services.<br>• Local preceptorship programme has great reviews by NQMs.<br>• Good chance of further training (i.e. cannulation, IV infusions, epidurals and suturing). | • Potential lack of support, not being supernumerary will make transition difficult.<br>• Women's attitudes towards young, newly qualified midwives.<br>• Unreasonable expectations of me. |

Now complete your own SWOT using the template provided (Activity 2.4). This can included in your professional portfolio (refer to Chapter 3, section "How to Create a Portfolio for Interviews and CPD") and taken to interview.

**ACTIVITY 2.4**

**My SWOT analysis**

| STRENGTHS (internal) | WEAKNESSES (internal) |
|---|---|
| | |
| **OPPORTUNITIES (external)** | **THREATS (external)** |
| | |

## STEP 2: EXPLORING OPTIONS

Having engaged in Activities 2.1–2.4 you should now feel able to answer some of the bigger questions (Figure 2.2). You can identify what you enjoy and whether you are looking for something old (an environment that is familiar) or something new (you are prepared to work in an unfamiliar area, on a rotation or speciality) and thought about the factors governing this (such as short-term expediency or a longer-term goal). Greater clarity can fuel your confidence to start researching options and help you draw up a list of avenues for investigation including the names of people who might help.

Refining your search from generic positions to posts in a discrete specialism may not have happened yet. Applications will often require a clear expression of interest in a designated area of practice. If you wish to work in general medicine, be prepared to have to make further choices regarding whether it is a medical assessment unit or a unit where the individual wards specialise in respiratory medicine or cardiology. An eating disorder or drug rehabilitation unit? Understanding how services are configured will help, so looking at the trust/employer's website is essential. However, if you do not want to be restricted, it is worth asking about the possibility of a rotational post. Rotational posts are attractive options to employees because you are not committing yourself indefinitely to working in one location; they offer the variety you are used to from programmed placements and can crystallise decisions long term.

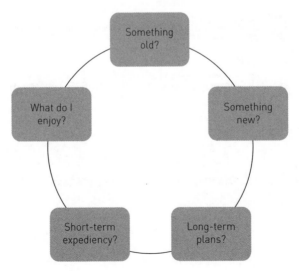

**FIGURE 2.2** The big questions!

From the employer's perspective, rotations arguably provide a more flexible workforce. Midwifery graduates might commence preceptorship programmes where they will be required to rotate through all the clinical areas. It is important to note that those contemplating becoming an independent midwife need to be aware that they would have to organise their own preceptorship. Under the One Year Guaranteed Job (OYJG) Scheme (NHS Education for Scotland 2015a) NQNs/NQMs in Scotland have the option of applying for the government internship programme. This offers rotational employment to consolidate and develop clinical experience on a fixed-term contract and supports completion of the Flying Start NHS® (NHS Education for Scotland 2015b).

Using the table provided below (Table 2.2), now complete the action plan (Activity 2.5).

**TABLE 2.2  Activity 2.5 career planning objectives: my next three steps**

| Action | How will you do it? | Timescale |
|---|---|---|
| Describe what you want to achieve as clearly as possible. | Will you need support? How will you evidence your success? | Set a date to complete this. |
| Example: *To identify suitable vacancies for paediatric nurses in ED in Leicester/ Northamptonshire* | • *Register with NHS Jobs and set up job alerts.*<br>• *Ask for help from Careers Destinations and staff on P5.*<br>• *Email alerts by end of week.* | *25 January* |
| 1. | | |
| 2. | | |
| 3. | | |

Taken from Careers Destinations University of Southampton (2014)

Creating an action plan will keep you focused, helps you set goals and time frames, benchmarks your progress and can ensure you achieve your goals. You should feel more in control. Remember to make your objectives SMART ones:

• Specific
• Measurable
• Achievable

- *Realistic*
- *Time* bound

In essence this process requires you to use the same skills that you employ when starting on an academic assignment, so be prepared for a few frustrations and those rewarding moments when your research yields useful results. The next sections look at where you can look and who you can ask for information.

## YOUR OWN NETWORK OF CONTACTS AND WORD OF MOUTH

This includes:

- Staff you have met on placement.
- Academic and research staff will have a very wide network and if they do not have a named contact in a locality will be able to refer to colleagues for advice.
- Visiting lecturers and clinical skills staff.
- Relatives, distant relatives, friends and friends of friends. Now is the time to re-ignite friendships through social media (Facebook) and let people know what your interests are and where you are looking for a job.

## WEBSITES

- NHS Jobs www.jobs.nhs.uk. Register and familiarise yourself with the layout and how to refine your search and set up job alerts so you are notified as soon as a job matching your preferences is advertised. Unless you are happy to move to a job anywhere in the UK do remember to select which geographical locations you want; otherwise your inbox will be inundated with emails.
- NHS Careers www.nhscareers.nhs.uk – the information service for NHS careers in England. It covers over 350 healthcare careers plus working and studying elsewhere in the UK. There is also a designated area on the website that provides advice for international healthcare professionals looking for work in the UK.
- Midwifery students should enrol on the Royal College of Midwives' official jobs board www.jobs.midwives.co.uk, an extensive resource with the facility to upload a CV and profile.
- Employer websites (statutory, independent, commercial, charitable, third sector and agencies).
- National, local and regional press (online and hard copy).

- The health sector pages on your university careers website. This will tell you where employers are likely to advertise.
- The university student portal; many universities have their own events and jobs listings.
- University websites. If you are looking at masters or doctoral (PhD) studies and learning beyond registration (LBR) opportunities, download and read a number of prospectuses. Enquire about recruitment processes and ask if there are open days where you can meet staff and current students.

## JOURNALS, BOOKS AND NOTICEBOARDS

- Career profiles in professional journals. These feature inspirational real-life stories and also will give you a name to contact if you want to find out more.
- Nursing and midwifery careers uncovered by Bird and Borrego (2010).
- Search professional journals and associated online websites:
  - *British Journal of Midwifery* info.britishjournalofmidwifery.com/
  - *Nursing Standard* www.nursing-standard-journal.co.uk through which you can also access the Royal College of Nursing jobs website www.rcnbulletinjobs.co.uk
  - *Nursing Times* www.nursingtimesjobs.com
- Noticeboards in health facilities.

## CAREERS FAIR

Your university and faculty will have a calendar of events such as careers fair and employer presentations to introduce undergraduates to job opportunities. You should also look out for local employer open days and recruitment events, national and regional jobs fairs such as the annual RCN Jobs Fair, the RCN annual congress and the RCM annual conference which have exhibition areas. Entry is often free and there may be a programme of employer presentations and seminars on topics like CVs and interview skills. Unless restrictions apply, all students, irrespective of whether or not they are finalists, should be encouraged to attend to gain early careers advice and experience a careers fair. That way, when they are final year students they know what to expect and how to work a jobs fair to their advantage.

Such events will give you a much wider appreciation of graduate employment opportunities, the job market, and help you to get ahead in planning your career. Careers fairs attract leading recruiters from a wide range of healthcare providers (trusts, the independent, voluntary and charitable sector organisations and recruitment agencies). They will be keen to meet you, discuss options and could potentially offer you an on-the-spot interview. There may also be companies offering "gap" placements; these can vary from 2 weeks to longer projects and add to your programmed work experience.

Here are some tips to help you get the most out of a jobs fair:

- Look at the list of exhibitors in advance so that you can research individual organisations and target your efforts and questions on the day at those who you are interested in applying to.
- Think carefully about your appearance; first impressions do count so an enthusiastic, well-presented student who can confidently walk up to a stranger and introduce himself or herself makes a good start. But this is not just about looking "employable"; it is also about your professionalism during conversations and in future correspondence. Recruiters will be imagining how you will be with their clients. Introductions are essential in the provision of compassionate patient-centred care so apply the #hellomynameis (Granger 2015) principle to every encounter.
- Sometimes there may be freebies (pens/sweets/post-its) to tempt people over to stands. Beware of these distractions for they can be used as a subtle means of distinguishing the focused, serious job hunter from the amateur collector!
- At a busy jobs fair you may have to wait your turn so you need to give yourself enough time for a meaningful discussion with those on your target list.
- Have a CV and/or business card with a QR (quick response) barcode ready to give a recruiter. The QR code can be linked to your personal webpage and CV.
- Write down the name of the person you spoke to and their contact details. Follow this up with an email. A recruiter who offers you their contact details and invites you to make an informal visit is showing you their keenness to progress an enquiry; it would be reasonable to expect a keen candidate to pursue this golden opportunity.

## INFORMAL VISITS

You do not need to wait until you are attending an interview to do more research into an organisation or area. If opportunity presents you could make an unsupervised visit to explore the general area and site; this can help resolve questions related to travel, parking and personal security. Respecting that access to clinical areas is restricted and you need permission to enter some sites, consider organising an "informal" visit so that, prior to application and interview, you can meet the manager, talk to staff and get a good "feel" for the clinical area. If there is the chance to speak with newly qualified staff on duty, ask them for their experiences of transition, available support and preceptorship.

In essence there is no such thing as an "informal" visit; how you set up and conduct yourself will be observed and noted by your hosts. This is both an information gathering and "marketing" exercise. The value of this is expanded upon in later sections (Chapter 4, section "The 'On the spot' Screening Interview" and Chapter 5, section "Background Research").

If you cannot find a vacancy in the specialism or locality where you want to work, another method is to write a speculative letter. The next section reviews the merits of this method and provides a template.

## THE SPECULATIVE LETTER

Speculative letters avoid the discomfort and awkward conversations associated with "cold calling" over the phone or in person. The applicant can choose who and when to make an approach. The idiom "speculate to accumulate" suggests an element of risk and chance and indeed the speculative letter is an enquiry about the chance of a job. There is always a risk too that the letter may not be answered. "Speculative" also means showing curiosity and interest so the letter is a formal expression of interest. It can have considerable impact if it is well composed, properly addressed to a named person and by good fortune happens to arrive when the employer is contemplating or actually advertising a role. It is not a speculative email; if you use email to send it, common courtesies apply in the email and the letter is an attachment. Box 2.2 offers an example which can be adapted to your own needs.

Recognising that a letter may be kept on file until such a time as a vacancy becomes available, a keen student might take this opportunity to ask for an informal visit anyway. If you are going to send out multiple enquiries do check the detail is correct in every instance. Sister Jackson at the Milford Unit will not be impressed to receive a letter addressed to her asking about vacancies in Redhill Community Services.

## MAKING SENSE OF JOB ADVERTISEMENTS

Some jobs may be ring-fenced for NQNs/NQMs and it will be made clear in the advertisement that the post is only for newly qualified staff. However, if it is a generic Band 5 and there are no restrictions

**BOX 2.2  Example of a speculative letter**

Dear Sister Jackson / Mrs Jackson

Ref: Vacancy enquiry

I am enquiring about possible future employment in a women's health environment and would be very grateful if you could consider me for a future staff nurse position on the Milford Unit.

In September I will be graduating from the University of Southampton with a Bachelor of Nursing Honours degree and Registered Nurse (Adult) status. I have been fortunate to have substantial experience in relevant placements during my training, including gynaecology, a recovery suite and a "well women" service in the community. My final placement will be in an acute medical admissions unit, which will enhance my management experience of acutely ill patients. In addition, I currently work a few hours each week as a healthcare assistant for NHS Professionals in Hampshire, which helps consolidate my training and broaden my experience.

From early on in my training, I realised that I gained greatest satisfaction from supporting women needing nurse-led care when receiving healthcare or enhancing their physical well-being. In particular I have developed an interest in using evidence to increase access to cancer screening services for women with learning difficulties; some of my academic work has focused on this important area of care. I am very keen to develop my skills and future practice in this field and contribute to high-quality and progressive nursing practice.

I realise that you are not currently advertising vacancies but would be most grateful if you would consider advising me when a suitable post becomes available. I enclose a current curriculum vitae for your perusal and would ask if you might keep it on file in the hope of a future vacancy. I can make myself available any time to visit informally if you think this might be helpful.

Thank you so much in anticipation of a future, favourable response.
Yours sincerely
Imogen Parker BN (Hons); RN (pending)
*Enc: Curriculum Vitae*

then this is open to all. Whilst employers may state that they would *"prefer"* candidates with post-qualification experience, any NQN/NQM can apply so do not let this statement deter you. Experience shows that final year students can successfully compete against qualified staff applying for a generic Band 5. Knowing that other applicants will have hours of registered practice to their name is unnerving to even the most confident, but that does not mean they are more employable and automatically qualify for the role. If students can demonstrate that they have the passion, willingness to learn and fresh ideas that an employer is looking for, they can secure jobs even though they may have less or sometimes no clinical experience in that area.

So if you have had relevant experience during a placement then you can use this to support your application. If you have not yet had experience, then think strategically. "Step 4: Gaining Experiences" suggests means by which you can augment your CV to make you worthy of consideration.

You might choose to apply for a number of vacancies (ring-fenced and generic). When you apply may be dependent on an organisation's recruitment cycle for NQN/NQMs posts so you need to ask recruiters about dates when job advertisements will be posted. Do not rely on word of mouth here; organisations may change the timings and, if inundated with responses, could bring forward the closing date for applications.

When a vacancy is advertised look carefully at the details and in particular note:

- How to apply
- Closing date and time
- The reference number and contact details
- Job description
- Type of contract (full- or part-time; flexible or fixed working hours)
- The required and desirable characteristics in the person specification
- Format of application
  - Online or hard copy?
  - Does it require just an application form, just a CV or both?
  - Does it require a covering letter?
- Offers of further advice, associated open days or pre-application visits

Print off the job advert/s and all the associated documentation. Use a highlighter pen to draw attention to key information and write down any questions you may have about the vacancy. It is advisable to contact the employer (HR department/clinical manager) if you are unsure about whether or not this is a vacancy that would be suitable for you. Before you make any call draft out your questions clearly so that you project yourself well during the conversation. How to compile an application is examined in depth in subsequent chapters.

## STEP 3: MAKING CHOICES

According to Gandhi (1869–1948), "Action expresses priorities". Making the right choice for you is difficult particularly if you have a number of possible options and competing priorities. What is right for one person will not be right for another so you need to think carefully, then decide and do what is ultimately right for you. This could mean you do not feel fully supported by significant others (family or friends) in this choice and this is something you need to reconcile and be comfortable with. You may want to work in a centre of excellence and this means moving away but there are emotional pressures to stay closer to home.

Identifying your priorities will help you to select which employer/s to target and to assess whether or not a job advertisement matches your needs. Now undertake Activity 2.6 (Table 2.3); for each of the suggested priorities ask yourself "Is this a priority when I am deciding which employer to apply to?" Tick those that are very important priorities. Then rank them in descending order, 1 being the most important priority with subsequent priorities having less significance.

| TABLE 2.3 Activity 2.6 my priorities for my first post are the following: | | |
|---|---|---|
| **Priorities** | **Tick those that are very important to you** | **Now rank these in order of priority (1 being most important)** |
| Consolidation of training | | |
| Supported transition to "first post" through preceptorship | | |
| Overall reputation of the organisation* | | |
| Culture of the organisation* | | |
| Content of work* | | |
| Rotation through different areas | | |
| Quality of staff already working for the employer* | | |
| Organisation's commercial and business performance | | |
| Promotion/career development prospects | | |

application. The core of a CV will not change; however, each version must be tailored to fit each job description and person specification.

Ask yourself, "Can I summarise myself in 140 characters?" With the advent of Twitter and social media sites such as LinkedIn, the traditional tabular CV has evolved into mini CV and micro resumé. These can have embedded QR codes that take a recruiter who is keen to learn more about a candidate to more detailed information. Many global companies now rely on social media platforms to post jobs and graduates tweet resumés (Zappe 2011; Bailey 2015). NQN/NQM recruitment in the UK is not yet at this point; if this is adopted as a way of recruiting healthcare staff, it needs to be well understood by applicants (refer also to Chapter 4, section "Social Networking and Lifestyle"). Inappropriate social media posts could close the door for an applicant even before the recruiter opens the tweet.

So with this in mind some might argue that the paper CV with its neat columns is nearing the end of its shelf life and question why we continue to encourage students to produce one. In reality there are a number of very good reasons why professional nurses and midwives need a contemporary CV. These are:

- To accompany speculative letters to potential employers or recruitment agencies
- To give out at careers/jobs fairs
- To populate the front pages of your personal professional portfolio (PPP)
- To demonstrate compliance with the NMC (2015b) requirements for renewing your registration and demonstrating your continuing fitness to practise:
  - the Continuing Professional Development (CPD) rules stipulate a minimum of 40 hours of CPD in 3 years; 20 of which must include participatory learning
  - a minimum total of 450 practice hours over 3 years for a nurse or a midwife
  - a minimum total of 900 practice hours over 3 years for those who have dual registration, that is, nurse and midwife (including nurse/specialist community public health nursing (SCPHN) and midwife/SCPHN) or dual fields, that is, adult and mental health. This is further split by registration into a minimum of 450 for nursing and 450 for midwifery
  - refer to www.nmc.org.uk/standards/revalidation/revalidation-guidance-and-resources
- To accompany research grant applications
- To meet institutional requirements, for example, university staff

When you complete an online application, a word-processed CV serves as an essential and central holding point for key information that you will harvest to populate the boxes. It is therefore worth investing time and effort in compiling your CV early on in the process, ideally *before* you need the information to meet a challenging deadline. A good time would be during year 2 of a 3-year programme or when academic pressures are at a low point and you can spend time seeking out and pulling together the information. The demographic information is not so much the issue; it is the detail around educational qualifications, dates and institutions that may not be on hand to students living away from home.

The finished item should be like its owner – that is professional, polished and perfect for the role. A CV outlines your accomplishments and when used well can set apart "a shining star" from a crowd of individuals, all of whom are exiting with the same professional registration. The recruiter may spend as little as 20–30 seconds scanning the CV that took you hours to compile, so it helps to abide by the 10 rules in Box 3.1 to impress and keep their attention.

---

### BOX 3.1 10 ways to make your CV work for you

1. Keep it brief and concise.
2. Keep it easy to read (use "plain English").
3. Keep to high-impact language.
4. Keep it on two pages of A4.
5. Keep the style clean, smart and simple:

   - Same font throughout (Arial or Times New Roman).
   - Embolden titles.
   - Adjust font size (14 for title, 12 for sub-headings and 11 for main text).
   - Use lists or tables to align content.
   - Use white space to separate sections and reduce overcrowding.
   - Avoid colour and images.

6. Keep content relevant to recipient.
7. Tell me about your most relevant achievements.
8. Tell me about your professional attributes.
9. Tell me about your potential.
10. Tell me you can do the job.

---

## CV TEMPLATES

Type in "CV template" in a search engine and you will find millions (literally) of examples. So where do you start? The Royal College of

Nursing (RCN) website has a CV builder which members can access. Innes' (2012a) book devoted to CVs provides a sample of formats, all of which are available as downloads. The commonality in all of these is the early inclusion of a "Professional Profile". This is a brief summary statement about you and should be between five and ten lines long. It sits immediately after the personal detail and if well constructed will entice the reader to spend more time looking through your CV.

Some content is essential and therefore by definition certain templates will work better for nursing and midwifery CVs. You may already have an old CV that needs updating. Whilst it is tempting to stick with a format you have used before, compare it with others such as the one used in this book and ask yourself, "Is the format I have used here fit for purpose?" Your institution may provide you with a completed example and a blank template for your use. Arguably you might feel that a template stifles your creative nature and you might worry that your CV will look like everyone else's. In defence of templates, they encourage a uniformity in approach through the use of tabulation and ensure the novice CV builder has not overlooked any essential information. The reader's eye is naturally drawn to information at the top and to the left-hand side of the page as opposed to the right. This is one very good reason to put the most important statement – your professional profile – first.

It is human nature to want to put in everything you have achieved, but the more achievements you have, the more ruthless you will have to be in order to keep to the standard two-page format. Once the structure and content are in place, you can experiment but make sure you do not sacrifice substance for looks.

Activity 3.1 is designed to help you understand the nuances of CV construction and to give an indication of the time you will need to set aside to compile your CV. In this exercise you will be critiquing a CV; not everything in Sophie's CV is poorly compiled, but some aspects could be significantly improved upon to make her achievements stand out.

This next section will take you step by step through the first draft of her CV, picking up on the detail.

## PERSONAL DETAILS

Aside from alignment (to left, right or centred), the recommended format for this introductory section is relatively plain. In Box 3.2 Sophie has made a few common errors.

## ACTIVITY 3.1

Read carefully through this CV and with a highlighter identify aspects that you think could be improved upon. Pay particular attention to layout, use of language, presentation of key achievements and note uncertainties that you need clarifying. Then compare your notes to the guidance.

### Curriculum Vitae (Draft 1)
#### Sophie Clare Jones
15a Captains House, Ocean Avenue, Southampton SO15 9RN

Hotleggs11@hotmail.com

Tel: 023 80 111 111; Mobile: 077712345678

LinkedIn: www.linkedin.com/XXXXX

## PROFESSIONAL QUALIFICATION
Registered Nurse (Adult)   NMC   Expected date: Sept 2015   PIN tba

## EDUCATION
**2012 – 2015**   **University of Southampton**
**Bachelor of Nursing (Hons) current average 74%**

**2010 – 2012**   **Waterside College**
GCE A Levels: Biology, Psychology and Mathematics

2005 – 2010   St Richard's Community School
GCSEs: 10 A* - C including Mathematics and English

## PROFESSIONAL SKILLS AND EXPERIENCE
**Oct – Dec 14**   **Placement 5, Acute Hospital**
- Worked as part of a multi-disciplinary team. Supported junior colleagues with client issues, including first- and second- year students.
- Admitted, assessed clients and prioritised care. Helped manage emergency admissions to the unit. Carried out clinical procedures in accordance with unit policy
- Attended an update on infection control run by the trust

**July – Aug 14**   **Placement 4, Community Placement, NHS Trust**
- Responded to needs and used my initiative when planning and delivering care in the clients' home
- Effectively managed a small caseload of clients

- Went to a support group for neurological conditions
- Gained lone worker experience
- Spent a week shadowing a community matron
- Ensured client records (manual and electronic) were maintained and reported in accordance with the trust policy

## EMPLOYMENT HISTORY
**Since 2013 - Healthcare Support Worker**
**NHS Professionals, Southampton**

## VOLUNTEER WORK
**Since 2012  Faculty of Health Sciences, University of Southampton**
- I am an ambassador for Health Sciences, visiting local colleges to talk about nursing

**Since 2011  Shelter, Southampton**
**Volunteer – Homeless Project Support**
- Regularly volunteer at weekends

## ADDITIONAL SKILLS
**Clinical** Completed all mandatory updates (moving and handling; Fire Safety; BLS; Trust Safeguarding)
**IT** Proficient in the use of Microsoft Office, email and Internet. Passed ECDL. I am trained in use of RIO client record system
**Driving** Full clean driving licence
**Languages** Conversational French; British Sign Language Level 1
**Interests** Open-water swimming, socialising, football, travel and reading

## INTERESTS AND ACTIVITIES
**Societies** Active member of the University of Southampton's Students Union Fundraising Committee. Recently did a charity bake-off in aid of UNICEF
A student member of the Royal College of Nursing
**Football** Member of Women's University 1st XI. Taken the responsibility for organising fixtures, liaising with other universities, arranging venues and transport and ensuring all players are aware of arrangements

## REFERENCES ARE AVAILABLE ON REQUEST

BOX 3.2 Sophie's draft

### Curriculum Vitae (Draft 1)
Sophie Clare Jones
15a Captains House, Ocean Avenue, Southampton SO15 9RN
Hotleggs11@hotmail.com
Tel: 023 80 111 111; Mobile: 077712345678
~~LinkedIn: www.linkedin.com/XXXXX~~

Sophie's CV is headed "Curriculum Vitae" or CV. This is unnecessary; the heading should comprise your first and last name only, in bold capitals. If your name does not clearly indicate your gender you can add your title (i.e. Mr, Mrs, Miss, etc.). All other details are superfluous and increase the risk of identity fraud. Your marriage status, religion, passport number or National Insurance number, your age and/or date of birth are not required, nor is a photograph. This advice complies with the Equality Act (Great Britain Parliament 2010). The inclusion of your nationality is only necessary if you are seeking sponsorship for a work permit.

### CONTACT DETAILS

These must be kept up to date; if you are nearing the end of your degree studies you should take into account the fact that your university email account may expire so using a suitable personal email account would be better. Likewise if you are likely to be moving out of student accommodation or relocating to another area but do not have a forwarding address to use, then use a permanent reliable address (i.e. parents' home) for the interim.

Sophie needs to reserve her hotleggs11@hotmail.com for personal correspondence. Better still replace it with a more staid and professional one. LinkedIn is a professional networking and profile tool; unless it adds any more substantive evidence of achievement there is little merit in having it as an extra point of contact. It is wise to give at least two contact phone numbers, usually home and mobile. And edit your voicemail message so that the caller gets a good first impression. A former student had her voicemail tampered with by flatmates. She was unaware of this until it was pointed out to her by her tutor who had rung several times. The voicemail message which said "I'm a Laaady!" (citing Robbie Williams in *Little Britain* 2009) gave the impression that this was an escort agency. You can imagine what an employer may have thought if this was their first impression of a prospective candidate.

The format is address, contact telephone numbers and then email. Sophie's amended personal and contact details should now look like this (see Box 3.3).

---

**BOX 3.3  Sophie's amended personal and contact details**

### Sophie Jones

15a Captains House, Ocean Avenue, Southampton SO15 9RN

Telephone: 023 80 111 111 (Home); 077712345678 (Mobile)

Sophie.Jones30@hotmail.com

---

## PROFESSIONAL PROFILE

You may have spotted that this vital section is absent from Sophie's CV (Box 3.4). If so, well done! The professional profile comes straight after personal and contact details and before professional education and qualifications sections.

---

**BOX 3.4  Where to position the professional profile**

### Curriculum Vitae (Draft 1)

Sophie Clare Jones

15a Captains House, Ocean Avenue, Southampton SO15 9RN

Hotleggs11@hotmail.com

Tel: 023 80 111 111; Mobile: 077712345678

LinkedIn: www.linkedin.com/XXXXX

PROFESSIONAL QUALIFICATION ⟶ No Professional Profile?

Registered Nurse (Adult)   NMC   Expected date: Sept 2015   PIN tba

---

A good professional profile can work like a good, firm introductory handshake. Aim for three sentences that will answer the following three questions:

Sentence 1: *Who are you?*
Sentence 2: *What are your skills?*
Sentence 3: *What do you want?*

Next look at Box 3.5 which outlines what Sophie could say about herself:

**BOX 3.5 Sophie's professional profile**

**Professional profile:**

A highly motivated adult nursing student with proven clinical, team-working and communication skills gained through three years of clinical placements and degree-level studies. An active and reflective learner, who is able to effectively manage a small caseload of clients and support junior students. Seeks the opportunity to further develop clinical, managerial and leadership skills as a Band 5 and become a significant asset to the medical unit at St Michael's NHS Foundation Trust.

You will notice that this section is a single paragraph rather than bullet points. Writing in the third person is recommended best practice (Innes 2012a) but this can be difficult. Dropping pronouns (I, we, you, he, she or they) altogether is much easier. So rather than "I am seeking the opportunity to further develop my clinical, etc." write "Seeks the opportunity to..." instead.

There are some common ideas that you will want to recycle. This is okay but you need to put them into your own words and edit them until you are confident that your profile sells you in a positive and meaningful way. What will you say about yourself? Now complete Activity 3.2.

**ACTIVITY 3.2**

**Writing your own professional profile**

1. Look at your last few assessments of practice reports.
2. Look at comments from one-to-one progress reviews with your tutor.
3. Make a list of the key attributes that your mentor has identified.
4. Look at the adjectives and phrases.
5. Is there anything else that you want the reader to know about you from the outset?
6. Now use these ideas to create your own professional profile.
7. Remember, no more than 10 lines max!

It would be no surprise if this activity has taken more time to complete than anticipated and is as frustrating as essay writing.

## EDUCATION AND QUALIFICATIONS

Sophie's professional education and qualifications are currently listed alongside her general education. This section needs reworking; you may have spotted some of the missing data as highlighted in Box 3.6 and have some questions about how to present this information.

---

**BOX 3.6  Sophie's draft professional education and qualifications**

### PROFESSIONAL QUALIFICATION

Registered Nurse (Adult)   NMC   Expected date: Sept 2015
PIN tba *is this ok?*

**EDUCATION**

| | |
|---|---|
| 2012 – 2015 | **University of Southampton**<br>**Bachelor of Nursing (Hons) current average 74%** |
| 2010 – 2012 | **Waterside College** *where is this?*<br>GCE A Levels: Biology, Psychology and Mathematics<br>*What grades?* |
| 2005 – 2010 | **St Richard's Community School** *where is this?*<br>GCSEs: 10 A* – C including Mathematics and English<br>*What grades?* |

---

Sophie has combined her professional education (degree) with her general education. This needs to be split; the recruiter will want to know that you have a relevant professional education, that is, degree in nursing or midwifery, post-graduate diploma, advanced diploma or diploma in nursing. They will be less concerned about qualifications that preceded it because these determined eligibility to commence your professional studies.

You will therefore need a general education section; however, this will come *after* professional experience and skills. By ordering the information this way you will not detract from the purpose which is to present your most relevant achievements first. You are not obliged to list grades or marks; however, Sophie is keen to flag up the fact that she is on track for a first-class honours degree classification so it is sensible to use this as a strong selling point. This is her "assessment average" across both practice and academic work so needs to be made a little clearer.

When you looked at Sophie's CV you may also have spotted incomplete addresses for her school and college and some missing grades. Gaps indicate one of three things, that is, poor attention to detail, poor time management or someone who is being economical with the truth. The latter is usually related to failure or embarrassment. Some students repeat exams in order to improve upon grades, take time out of study or, as mature students, after a career break or family return to study in order to get the qualifications required to enrol on a degree in midwifery or nursing. The dates will give the reader some indication of your educational journey and your determination to achieve.

Under professional education and qualifications you need to indicate:

- Dates, name of institution and degree programme title
- Date of registration/expiry date. If you are yet to qualify this should be the anticipated date
- Name of qualification
- Which part of the register you are on (adult, learning disabilities, midwife, mental health or child)
- Name of regulator, that is, Nursing and Midwifery Council (abbreviate to NMC)
- PIN or PIN to be advised (TBA)

Taking this into account, we would advise Sophie to amend this section accordingly (Box 3.7).

---

**BOX 3.7 Sophie's amended professional education and qualifications**

### PROFESSIONAL EDUCATION AND QUALIFICATION

| | |
|---|---|
| **Sept 2012 – Sept 2015** | University of Southampton<br>Bachelor of Nursing (Hons) current assessment average 74% |
| **Expected Sept 2015** | Registered Nurse (Adult)   NMC   PIN TBA |

**PROFESSIONAL SKILLS AND EXPERIENCE – see section "Professional skills and experience"**

**GENERAL EDUCATION**

| | |
|---|---|
| **2010 – 2012** | **Waterside College, Plymouth, Devon**<br>3 A Levels: Biology (A), Psychology (B), Mathematics (B) |
| **2005 – 2010** | **St Richard's Community School, Saltash, Devon**<br>10 GCSEs: A* – C including Mathematics (A*) and English (A) |

If you have dual registration, the most recent qualification is cited first. As your career progresses and you acquire additional qualifications you need to add these to your CV. There are three categories of NMC recordable qualifications; these are specialist practitioners on NMC-approved programmes, nurse prescribers and teachers.

The section on general education will contain all your other qualifications, again working in reverse chronological order so the most recent (i.e. A levels, access course, first degree, etc.) will come first.

## PROFESSIONAL SKILLS AND EXPERIENCE

Sophie has tried hard to summarise her achievements and is not using any pronouns which is good, but this is the section she needs most help to get right. Again the rule of thumb is to list placements in descending order (most recent first). Do remember to add in additional electives, practice development experience (PDE), Erasmus exchange visits or internships. Space is at a premium so you will need to make educated decisions about the worth of including first and second year placements. If an earlier placement is one you wish to return to as an NQN/NQM, then this should be included because you can emphasise what you learnt and what you will bring to the role.

Fundamentally you want to show the reader you are ready to qualify and have the skill set and attitude they are looking for. This you need to do by describing what you did and importantly your achievements. Let's look at Sophie's first draft summary in Box 3.8 of her achievements in Placement 5.

---

**BOX 3.8 Sophie's draft Placement 5 achievements**

Oct – Dec 14     Placement 5, Acute Hospital

- Worked as part of a multi-disciplinary team. Supported junior colleagues with client issues, including first and second year students.
- Admitted, assessed clients and prioritised care. Helped managed emergency admissions to the unit.
- Carried out clinical procedures in accordance with unit policy.
- Attended an update on infection control run by the trust.

---

Now compare this with a revised version in Box 3.9. Adjustments to the layout have created more space for essential detail. Here the vocabulary is varied and there is greater use of action verbs and adjectives to make it a stronger, more engaging read. The key skills she wants the recruiter to see are at the top and clinical procedures are itemised.

---

**BOX 3.9 Sophie's revised Placement 5 achievements**

Oct – Dec 2014    Placement 5, Acute Medical Admissions Unit, University Hospital X NHS Trust

- Became competent in admitting, assessing and prioritising the care of the acutely unwell patient
- Effectively managed a bay of six patients, monitoring, delivering and coordinating their care
- Practised junior management skills, delegated responsibilities appropriately to colleagues
- Developed strong working relationships with the multi-disciplinary team including ambulance service
- Efficiently organised and safely transferred patients to other units
- Frequently acted as second nurse on drug rounds to develop proficiencies in medicines management and use of e-prescribing software
- Helped orientate and supported first- and second-year nursing and medical students during their placements
- Became proficient in complex nursing skills (i.e. female catheterisation; NEWS; SBAR) in accordance with trust policy and best practice standards
- Participated in an excellent trust update on infection control, reviewed current evidence base and recommended best practice in relation to hand hygiene

---

The vocabulary is very important and needs to be varied to avoid repetition. You will need a list of action verbs and positive adjectives to describe yourself. Sophie is evidently safe. She refers to trust policy and best practice. In the revised version she tells us exactly what she gained personally from participating in the "excellent trust update on infection control". This contrasts the very passive, unengaged tone adopted in the draft which refers to attendance but does not acknowledge the learning achieved.

On the revised complete CV on pages 55–57 you will see that Placement 5 has likewise been embellished and an elective experience added to demonstrate additional skills like negotiation and self-directed learning.

To stretch yourself, try the exercise in Activity 3.3.

## ACTIVITY 3.3

### The alphabet brain game

This can be done on your own or as a fun group activity with colleagues. Work your way through the alphabet and write down the words.

- Two action verbs for each letter. So A is for "analysed" and "assessed", B is for... etc.
- Now repeat the same for positive adjectives. For example, E is for "effective" and "enthusiastic", F is for "flexible" and "fastidious", etc.
- You might want to raise the bar to see just how many you can identify for each letter of the alphabet.

You have just created a great resource.

If you are short on time you can refer to a dictionary or a thesaurus – accessible on the review bar of most computer programmes or simply type in "action verbs" on a search engine. There are numerous examples such as University of Victoria's (2011) list of action verbs available from www.uvic.ca/coopandcareer/assets/docs/corecompetencies/Action_verb_list_infosheet.pdf.

It is important to be truthful and you must have evidence to support any statement you make. The best record of your placement successes to date will be found in your assessment of practice portfolio so you now need to refer back to your mentor reports, self-assessments and reflections. These contemporary accounts should provide a wealth of evidence you can use to compile a compelling list of attainment. The most important achievement should be at the top of the list.

The other key resources you need to refer to when compiling your CV are the following:

- Job vacancy advertisement
- Job description
- Person specification
- Set of organisation's values (see Chapter 4, section "Values-Based Recruitment (VBR)")

In Chapter 4, section "Essential Skills" there is an exercise based around a Band 5 job description. Within the job description and person specification there will be plenty of action verbs and positive adjectives about the role and characteristics of the ideal candidate. If you have not already done this exercise, consider doing this now.

## GENERAL EDUCATION

This section sits after professional skills and experience. The content was discussed in section "Education and Qualifications".

## EMPLOYMENT HISTORY

Again you need to provide information about your most recent first. It should be a comprehensive list of employment to date. When you saw Sophie's you might have asked yourself "Is this all?" It tells the reader nothing about what Sophie actually does in this role, nor what she has gained from this experience by way of transferable skills that would interest a prospective employer (Box 3.10).

---

**BOX 3.10 Sophie's draft employment history**

EMPLOYMENT HISTORY

| Since 2013 | **Healthcare Support Worker NHS Professionals, Southampton** |

Is this all?

---

Candidates with a long career history will have to use the available space wisely. Too much detail about previous jobs can unbalance a CV so it is important to be concise. Conversely, those with little or no work experience will have to make more of any unpaid or temporary work. Sophie can therefore include her very part-time waitressing job. The essential details are:

- Start date: Month/year
- End date: Month/year
- Title of role
- Employer's name and location
- And importantly, a description of the main duties and responsibilities

Continue to focus on the language and use action verbs to emphasise transferable skills such as problem-solving, responsibility and customer service experience. You can refer to the trust/organisation's values for inspiration (see Chapter 4, section "Values-Based Recruitment (VBR)"). Box 3.11 contains Sophie's revised employment history.

**BOX 3.11 Sophie's revised employment history**

## EMPLOYMENT HISTORY

### Jun 2013 – date Healthcare Support Worker NHS Professionals, Southampton

- Readily adapt to new settings, situations and practices
- Support patients with personal care and nutritional needs

### Jun 2010 – date   Waitress, Bill's Diner, Saltash, Devon

- Greeting and serving customers; keeping the tearooms clean and tidy
- Achieved Food Hygiene Certificate 2011

You are not required to, nor should you, provide information pertaining to salary or reason for leaving. If there are gaps, and in many instances there will be, you need to be prepared for a question about this at interview. There are gaps for legitimate reasons such as undertaking further study, caring for a dependant (child or elderly parent) or travel. A brief entry will suffice and is considered to be better than an unexplained gap (Innes 2010a). Unemployment and ill health, whilst good reasons in themselves, are more difficult to present so are best left off to be discussed, if raised, at interview.

## VOLUNTEER WORK

If you do not currently volunteer, perhaps now is the time to look for suitable opportunities. Local organisations may be in need of assistance. Volunteer work does not have to relate solely to charitable activities; it includes any unpaid activity such as youth or faith work, sports coaching, befriending services or assisting as a parent in a school activity. Employers like to see individuals contributing to their communities. Often students worry about being tied to a regular commitment and competing academic and placement demands. Some schemes may be looking for short-term volunteer helpers or ad hoc assistance. University student services or Students Union will have information about a range of local projects and can match your availability, interests and skill set accordingly. It is not unusual for a volunteering experience to open more doors and opportunities for participants.

The section on Sophie's draft CV presents her as a student who the faculty view as a good ambassador; in addition Sophie is a regular volunteer at a local homeless project (Box 3.12).

**BOX 3.12 Sophie's draft volunteer work**

**VOLUNTEER WORK**

| | |
|---|---|
| **Since 2012** | **Faculty of Health Sciences, University of Southampton** |

- I am an ambassador for Health Sciences, visiting local colleges to talk about nursing

**Since 2011**   **Shelter, Southampton**
**Volunteer – Homeless Project Support**

- Regularly volunteer at weekends Doing what?

With slight adjustment to the wording, to emphasise the achievement and keep the format consistent (i.e. remove pronoun "I"), Sophie can make more of the skills she has acquired (Box 3.13). Rather than using the term "regularly" which is non-specific, she stipulates that her commitment is two days a month.

**BOX 3.13 Sophie's amended volunteer work**

**VOLUNTEER WORK**

**April 2014 – date**     **Faculty of Health Sciences, University of Southampton**

- Chosen as an ambassador for Health Sciences; visited local colleges to give presentations to students considering a career in nursing

**May 2011 – date**     **Shelter, Southampton. Volunteer with Homeless Support Project**

- Voluntary work (two days a month)
- Developed an ability to build relationships with vulnerable individuals
- Increased confidence to deal with challenging situations, that is, intoxicated clients

## ADDITIONAL SKILLS

This section is where you record all your achievements. Have a look at Sophie's list (Box 3.14); many of these will be ones that you too have acquired over your 3- or 4-year programme. A driving licence may be a prerequisite for some roles such as community posts so there is a designated space for this. It is important to separate additional skills from interests and hobbies.

Using the same headings that Sophie has will help you order the contents. All students will have undertaken mandatory training but do not forget to include extras like safeguarding updates and extra-curricular modules that show you are a motivated learner.

---

**BOX 3.14 Sophie's draft additional skills section**

**ADDITIONAL SKILLS**

| | |
|---|---|
| **Clinical** | Completed all mandatory updates (moving and handling; Fire Safety; BLS; Trust Safeguarding) DATES? |
| **IT** | Proficient in the use of Microsoft Office, email and Internet. Passed ECDL. I am trained in use of RIO client record system |
| **Driving** | Full clean driving licence |
| **Languages** | Conversational French; British Sign Language Level 1 |
| **Interests** | Open-water swimming, socialising, football, travel and reading |

---

Sophie's list could be neatened up, abbreviations written out in full and there is essential detail missing. She is evidently a sociable person so there is no need to put in "socialising" (see Box 3.15).

---

**BOX 3.15 Sophie's amended additional skills section**

**ADDITIONAL SKILLS**

| | |
|---|---|
| **Clinical** | Mandatory moving and handling update September 2013; Fire Safety update October 2013; Basic Life Support update July 2014; Trust Safeguarding update August 2014 |
| **IT** | Passed ECDL (2012). Proficient in the use of Microsoft Office, email and Internet. Trained in use of RIO client record system (2014) |
| **Driving** | Full clean driving licence |
| **Languages** | Conversational French; British Sign Language Level 1 (2014) |

---

## INTERESTS AND ACHIEVEMENTS

Here you can list membership of professional bodies such as RCN, RCM or UNISON. Students who get involved in student-staff liaison roles as representatives for their cohort or in the Students Union demonstrate a level of involvement that sets them apart from their counterparts. The skills you develop such as organising and chairing meetings, presenting feedback and influencing change are highly transferable.

Recruiters want well-rounded, personable employees so think carefully about how you can make your personality jump off the page. Each interest you include serves a purpose and you may be asked about it at interview. Have a look at Sophie's entries in Box 3.16. She is active in the Students Union and has a breadth of interesting hobbies, including a team sport and several means of relaxation.

---

**BOX 3.16 Sophie's draft interests and achievements**

**INTERESTS AND ACTIVITIES** *Use bullet points. Summarise!*

| | |
|---|---|
| **Societies** | Active member of the University of Southampton's Students Union Fundraising Committee. Recently did a charity bake-off in aid of UNICEF <br> A student member of the Royal College of Nursing |
| **Football** | Member of Women's University 1st XI. Taken the responsibility for organising fixtures, liaising with other universities, arranging venues and transport and ensuring all players are aware of arrangements |

---

Again this needs sharpening to maximise effect (Box 3.17) because recruiters will not linger.

---

**BOX 3.17 Sophie's amended interests and achievements**

**INTERESTS AND ACTIVITIES**

- Active member of the University of Southampton's Students Union Fundraising Committee. Recently organised a "Bake Off" which raised £500 for UNICEF
- Student member of the Royal College of Nursing
- Football (played for Women's University 1st XI; fixtures coordinator)
- Open-water swimming for relaxation
- Films and reading poetry

---

## REFERENCES

Job offers will be subject to the outcome of health assessment and receipt of satisfactory references. To this end, candidates will be asked to provide the names of at least two referees, a clinical referee and an academic referee. Occasionally they may also require a character or personal referee. Sophie's first draft stated that "REFERENCES ARE AVAILABLE ON REQUEST".

This is fine; details arguably take up valuable space (Innes 2010a). This is information for the application form so providing you have all of this information ready you do not need to include it on the CV.

## HOW TO IDENTIFY SUITABLE REFEREES

Think carefully about who is the right person to be your referee. Make a list of people you might approach. Ask yourself:

- Is this person suitably qualified?
- Is this someone whose opinion and authority will be respected by an employer?
- Are there other reasons why I have chosen them? If so what are these?

Being a referee gives those who have been involved in your supervision and successes the chance to make commendations and help you into employment. Tutors and mentors regard it as a professional privilege. That said, everyone has the right to refuse to act as a referee. Very few do and if they do they should justify this decision. To this end and to avoid embarrassment, it is a common courtesy and wise to approach people in advance to gain permission before you cite them as a referee. The guiding principles for any reference are that it cannot be used to defame a person and should either state only positives or nothing at all. References should comply with legislation, namely:

- Data Protection Act (Information Commissioner's Office (ICO) 1998) and Subject Access right in relation to references (ICO 2014)
- Equality Act (Great Britain Parliament 2010) for the UK (excluding Northern Ireland)
- In Northern Ireland the Disability Discrimination Act (1995 Northern Ireland Government) and Disability Discrimination (NI) Order 2006 (DDO) (Northern Ireland Government)

## THE ACADEMIC REFEREE

This should be your academic tutor who is best placed to comment on your progress and capabilities. If they have supported you over the full course of a programme they will have witnessed your professional transformation and have discussed your career choices with you. This will help them to tailor their comments to your application, for example, "Debra's ambition is to work in the community". The more information you provide, the more individual the reference. In the event that you have had a recent change of tutor, you should ask your current tutor's advice. They may need to consult with colleagues and records or feel that the former tutor would be better/best equipped to provide this information.

There is no one set format for responding to a reference request; institutions usually have an agreed end-of-programme reference template which is completed by the supervising academic. Institutions often issue guidelines about what can and cannot be stated in line with legislation. The future employer may also request a computer-generated transcript of training which would include detail such as grades and pass/fail outcomes for modules. This would be necessary if a candidate is applying to work abroad or continue in higher education. You may be charged for this service.

The end-of-programme summary reference will state your academic and practice attainment to date and could include pertinent extracts from assessment of practice feedback. This is a legal, confidential document so must be factually accurate at the time it is issued. An academic referee cannot provide information on sickness or absence. If you have yet to complete and satisfy the NMC requirements for registration, it will state exactly that. Your academic tutor may ask for your input or permission, particularly if there is a perceived benefit in sharing certain detail, such as the need for reasonable adjustment (i.e. for dyslexia) with the potential employer. The reference will not usually elude to the reason for a delay in completion, for example, when a programme has been extended to allow for further attempts at unpassed assessments or due to unforeseen circumstances such as a bereavement. However, should you decide that there is no benefit to divulging such information, you need to be aware that an employer may ask you why you did not complete at the predicted time.

If a candidate has been offered a job but cannot subsequently complete on time because of academic failure, they should be quick to notify the employer and be honest and explain why. The employer may want to contact the referee (academic tutor) for reassurances, to work with the institute and, if they are able to keep the job offer open, negotiate a later start date. The enquiry is often handled by the head of programme who manages the assessment process. In our experience, employers are genuinely reluctant to lose any candidates who excelled at interview and are otherwise safe in practice. However, if the reason for non-completion is due to a practice referral and the need for additional support, then an employer could reasonably withdraw their job offer.

You will need to submit their full name, including title (Mr, Mrs, Dr, Prof, etc.), full address and contact numbers (email and telephone).

Attention to detail is essential; if there are any inaccuracies it could result in difficulties obtaining a reference. If you have space and choose to include the names of referees on your CV adopt the format used in Box 3.18. The inclusion of their title is usually sufficient to denote whether it is an academic or clinical referee.

---

**BOX 3.18 How to set out references at the end of the CV**

**REFERENCES**

Eileen Reed (Mrs)
Lecturer in Nursing
Faculty of Health Sciences
Bldg 22
University Campus
Anytown
SO1 61J
Tel: 012 80 222 333
Email: eileen.reed@anytown.ac.uk

Archie Roberts
Senior Staff Nurse
Acute Medical Assessment Unit
University Hospital X NHS Trust
Hamble Road
Anytown
SO19 10Q
Tel: 012 80 123 123
Email: Archie.roberts@uhx.nhs.uk

---

## THE CLINICAL REFEREE

This usually creates a dilemma; by the point you complete your programme you will have had at least six different practice placements and been mentored by six or more mentors and their respective buddies. The quality of the mentor-student relationship will have been variable and will have undoubtedly affected your thoughts on the overall experience and your learning. You may be drawn back to individuals because you feel you had a good relationship; conversely you are less likely to choose someone who you felt was overly critical of you in their mentor report.

The choice might seem obvious; you are applying for a vacancy in an area where you had a placement in Year 1, so you think about approaching the person who was your mentor back then. There are several key questions to ask yourself here; one is "Will they remember me?" bearing in mind that two years and many more students have passed through the placement. The second is "Does this person know me as I am now, that is, as a final year student?" If you left a lasting and positive impression then it is possible that you are remembered; however, the answer to the second question will be "no". Even if you have subsequently returned to do regular bank work, be careful because you are in a different role and one which does not incorporate summative assessment against final year competencies.

The best placed person will be one of your most recent mentors, ideally from the first placement in your final year where staff will be judging you in your capacity as a senior student, nearing the point of transition. Fundamentally you want someone you can trust to write a fair and hopefully "glowing" reference that will assure an employer that they have chosen wisely. Likewise you will need all their contact details and a work email address for correspondence. It is not usual for people to provide home contact details, unless they are going to be off work for any length of time (for example on study or maternity leave) and are willing to be contacted.

## THE PERSONAL REFERENCE OF GOOD CHARACTER

It is less usual for employers to request a personal character reference on standard employment checks. Under certain circumstances such as passport and visa applications, work permits, tenancy agreements or court proceedings you may be required to cite someone for this purpose. This type of reference allows the referee to comment on personal attributes such as honesty and integrity. You would not use a relative or partner; instead you would choose a friend or associate who has known you for a reasonable number of years (at least 5 years). It is better if they have professional standing in the community, for example, a teacher, a midwife or nurse, a religious leader or a lawyer. It may be someone you have worked with in a community capacity such as a youth leader.

If your mentor needs a template for a reference there are a range of reference templates available from www.businessballs.com/references lettersamples.htm.

### THE FINISHED ARTICLE

Invite a critical friend, tutor or designated careers adviser to critique your CV. Include your name and page number at the foot of each page. Once you have finalised the content, print out copies on good-quality A4 paper. You can use white, ivory or cream and should print only on one side. Place the unfolded sheets in a plastic wallet to keep them pristine. Refer to the complete revised CV for Sophie Jones on pages 55–57.

Remember that the CV is not a static tool. Each time you decide to send out a copy, revisit the content and adjust it so that it matches the purpose and the audience for whom it is intended. If you do declare your commitment to working for a particular organisation, make sure you change the name before you send it to another. It might seem obvious but we are only human and, when under pressure, mistakes happen.

## SOPHIE JONES

15a Captains House, Ocean Avenue, Southampton SO15 9RN
Telephone: 023 80 111 111 (Home); 077712345678 (Mobile)
Sophie.Jones30@hotmail.com

### PROFESSIONAL PROFILE

A highly motivated adult nursing student with proven clinical, team-working and communication skills gained through 3 years of clinical placements and degree-level studies. An active and reflective learner, who is able to effectively manage a small caseload of clients and support junior students. Seeks the opportunity to further develop clinical, managerial and leadership skills as a Band 5 and become a significant asset to the medical unit at St Michael's NHS Foundation Trust.

### PROFESSIONAL EDUCATION AND QUALIFICATION

**Sept 2012 – Sept 2015**   University of Southampton
Bachelor of Nursing (Hons) current assessment average 74%

**Expected Sept 2015**   Registered Nurse (Adult)   NMC   PIN TBA

### PROFESSIONAL SKILLS AND EXPERIENCE

**Oct – Dec 2014**   **Placement 5, Acute Medical Admissions Unit, University Hospital X NHS Trust**

- Became competent in admitting, assessing and prioritising the care of the acutely unwell patient
- Effectively managed a bay of six patients, monitoring, delivering and coordinating their care
- Practised junior management skills, delegated responsibilities appropriately to colleagues
- Developed strong working relationships with the multi-disciplinary team including ambulance service
- Efficiently organised and safely transferred patients to other units
- Frequently acted as second nurse on drug rounds to develop proficiencies in medicines management and use of e-prescribing software
- Helped orientate and supported first and second year nursing and medical students during their placements

- Became proficient in complex nursing skills (i.e. female catheterisation, NEWS, SBAR and handovers) in accordance with trust policy and best practice standards
- Participated in an excellent trust update on infection control, reviewed current evidence base and recommended best practice in relation to hand hygiene

**July – Aug 2014**       **Placement 4, Community Nursing Team, Test NHS Trust**

- Effectively managed a small caseload of clients and coordinated their care
- Used my initiative when encountering challenges (i.e. non-healing wounds; concerns about client self-medication skills and safe guarding of vulnerable clients)
- Gained substantial lone worker experience and an understanding of the associated health and safety issues
- Participated in a support group for clients with degenerative neurological conditions
- Time with the community matron and Rapid Response Team increased understanding of how the virtual ward can manage people in their own home
- Ensured client records (manual and electronic) were maintained and reported in accordance with the trust policy, NMC standards and the Data Protection Act (1998)

**May 2014**       **Elective placement HMP X, Devon**

- This 3-week placement was organised independently and was based around a set of personal learning objectives, negotiated with the healthcare team at the prison
- It provided an insight into prison nursing, assessment and treatment of primary and urgent unscheduled care needs (minor injuries to life-threatening emergencies such as hanging)
- Increased awareness of substance misuse and associated mental health issues, predicting and managing aggression/violence and medicines management in prisons

## GENERAL EDUCATION

**2010 – 2012**       **Waterside College, Plymouth, Devon**
3 A Levels: Biology (A), Psychology (B), Mathematics (B)

**2005 – 2010**       **Richard's Community School, Saltash, Devon**
10 GCSEs: A* – C including Mathematics (A*) and English (A)

## EMPLOYMENT HISTORY

**Jun 2013 – date**      **Healthcare Support Worker NHS Professionals, Southampton**

- Readily adapt to new settings, situations and practices
- Support patients with personal care and nutritional needs

**Jun 2010 – date**      **Waitress, Bill's Diner, Saltash, Devon**

- Greeting and serving customers; keeping the tearooms clean and tidy
- Achieved Food Hygiene certificate 2011

## VOLUNTEER WORK

**April 2014 – date**      **Faculty of Health Sciences, University of Southampton**

- Chosen as an ambassador for Health Sciences; visited local colleges to give presentations to students considering a career in nursing

**May 2011 – date**      **Shelter, Southampton. Volunteer with Homeless Support Project**

- Voluntary work (two days a month)
- Developed an ability to build relationships with vulnerable individuals
- Increased confidence to deal with challenging situations, that is, intoxicated clients

## ADDITIONAL SKILLS

**Clinical**      Mandatory moving and handling update September 2013; Fire Safety update October 2013; Basic Life Support update July 2014; Trust Safeguarding update August 2014

**IT**      Passed ECDL (2012). Proficient in the use of Microsoft Office, email and Internet. Trained in use of RIO client record system (2014)

**Driving**      Full clean driving licence

**Languages**      Conversational French; British Sign Language Level 1 (2014)

## INTERESTS AND ACTIVITIES

- Active member of the University of Southampton's Students Union Fundraising Committee. Recently organised a "Bake Off" which raised £500 for UNICEF
- Student member of the Royal College of Nursing
- Football (played for Women's University 1st XI; fixtures coordinator)
- Open-water swimming for relaxation
- Films and reading poetry

REFERENCES ARE AVAILABLE ON REQUEST

## COMPLETING APPLICATIONS

This process is critical in securing an interview. There are benefits to approaching this like a military operation leaving nothing to chance. The key driver will be the closing date so you need to plan to have all the paperwork complete well in advance. If it is a paper application remember to allocate additional time to mitigate against postal strikes or delays – do not relay on internal mail. If there is any uncertainty it is worth paying for a track and trace recorded delivery service.

NHS Jobs and other larger employers will require you to initially register online before selecting individual jobs. Always make a note of your ID or reference number. Online applications can be saved in draft form and amended until you are ready to submit. It is helpful to download a blank copy of the form and with a highlighter mark any sections that require information you do not have immediately to hand. Paper applications can be photocopied so you can make sure your answers fit into the blank spaces before you transpose the information into the top copy.

In both instances the devil is in the detail and this is what the employer wants to see. They will screen to see you:

- Can follow each instruction to the letter, that is, BLOCK capitals where requested
- Complete every section
- Write neatly and legibly/type carefully
- Adhere to word-count restrictions
- Spell accurately
- Use grammar and punctuation correctly
- Are accurate with dates, names, places, etc.
- Sign and date all forms as indicated

You will use the CV to populate your application form with the personal data. There will be a dedicated section for supporting information (see section "Personal Statements" on pages 62–68). Online applications do not have spellcheck facilities so you will have to spellcheck before copying and pasting from a word-processed document into the application itself.

In Box 3.19 is a checklist that pulls together all the actions you will need to take in readiness for submitting your application. It is here as an aide-memoire – under pressure it is easy to forget a crucial part of the process.

BOX 3.19 **Application To-Do List**

| Action: | Tick upon completion |
|---|---|
| Update my CV | |
| Make a note of the job advertisement number and closing date for applications | |
| Download all the associated documents | |
| Contact organisation by phone or email | |
| Carefully read and follow the application instructions | |
| Make a note of the key contact | |
| Ask for an informal visit | |
| Read and highlight key words in the advert, person specification and job description | |
| Make a list of the knowledge and skills required | |
| Write personal statement | |
| Plan the evidence you will use to demonstrate achievement of the necessary skills and attributes | |
| Ask a critical friend, tutor or careers adviser to proofread your personal statement | |
| Complete application form, including your personal statement | |
| Proofread your application several times | |
| Ask a critical friend to proofread your application (especially spelling, grammar and punctuation) | |
| Submit final document in advance of closing date | |
| Print off your own copy of the application form | |
| Make a note of the reference and your ID | |
| Always follow up your application | |

## INTEGRITY IN APPLICATIONS

Throughout the process your honesty and integrity should be beyond reproach. False claims or the falsification of records will jeopardise job offers and potentially a career. However, there may be potentially difficult subjects such as ill health, disability, criminal convictions or work permits that some candidates will need to discuss with an employer. Chapter 4, section "Applications, Interview Conduct and the Law" is all about Employment Law. The NHS operates a Guaranteed Interview Scheme (NHS Jobs 2014) which entitles an applicant with a disability to a guaranteed interview, providing they meet the minimum criteria within the person specification for the particular vacancy. The advert and application form should have the "positive about disabled people" symbol (with two ticks) on adverts and application forms (Her Majesty's Government 2014). If you have a disability and wish to be considered under the Guaranteed Interview Scheme, you must indicate this under the relevant section of the NHS Jobs application form.

A careers adviser will be able to give you confidential advice on how to manage uncomfortable conversations. Boxes 3.20–3.23 contain situations that are not uncommon and a reply from a recruiter as to a sensible way forward around disclosure.

### BOX 3.20 Tom's story

Tom (24) is soon to qualify as a RN Child. Eight years ago when he was 16 and at school he received a caution from the police for shoplifting a pack of batteries. The shopkeeper did not prosecute, but Tom was not a minor so the caution went on his record. He is not proud of this. He declared this at interview for the programme 3 years ago but is worried his caution will appear again on future DBS checks. What should he do?

**Our recruiter says**, "I think it is best to be honest and upfront with these issues. Cautions may still appear on DBS checks despite them often stating that they are removed after a certain time. It is better to declare any cautions."

### BOX 3.21 Amy's story

Amy is a midwifery student. In Year 2 she had to suspend her studies because her father died after a short illness. Subsequently she suffered from depression and had counselling. After 9 months she was well enough to return and has successfully completed all her assessments. Her programme was extended by 9 months so she will qualify much later than her counterparts. She is worried that her mental health problems will go against her. When and what should she tell a prospective employer?

**Our recruiter says**, "Qualifying later than anyone else would raise questions but if the reasons are declared it should make no difference to securing a post. Again, be open and honest. Amy would need to be aware of her own health and know when to seek help if she feels her health is deteriorating, and this is perhaps something to be shared at interview if Amy feels comfortable to do so. Recruiters are not allowed to ask about sickness."

---

## BOX 3.22  Vicky's story

Vicky is also about to qualify as an RN Mental Health. During her final placement with a community mental health team she went to visit a vulnerable client. She found the client dead from a suspected overdose of a prescribed medication. Vicky was asked to provide a statement to the police. The investigation is ongoing and she has been asked to attend court. She wants to work for the same trust when she qualifies but is not sure if, when and what she should tell a prospective employer.

**Our recruiter says**, "Vicky needs to be truthful and tell her employer all the details of the investigation if she is allowed to do so at interview. It must be very stressful to have found a client dead and it may affect interview performance knowing the court case is imminent. Interview panels will take this into consideration. It should not affect Vicky in her pursuit of a post within the same organisation."

---

## BOX 3.23  Mike's story

Mike is an extremely hard-working and conscientious student who has had extra support for his dyslexia. He qualifies for reasonable adjustments, which means extra time for exams and software to help with his studies. In practice staff have usually been understanding, but there have been the odd occasions when people have judged him "unfairly" for his disability. He is worried that a prospective employer might do the same. What should he do?

**Our recruiter says**, "Mike will have developed his own strategies to manage his dyslexia over time. It is important that recruiters are aware of his dyslexia as reasonable adjustments may need to be made within the area he has chosen to work. Many NHS organisations have staff employed with dyslexia, which is successfully managed by both the person and the organisation. If Mike feels that he is being judged unfairly for his disability by any member of staff, he must escalate this immediately as no employer will tolerate this behaviour and will treat this as a very serious offence which would lead to dismissal of that staff member."

## PERSONAL STATEMENTS

The personal statement again needs to be tailored to an individual application. It comprises information that will occupy the section titled "Additional Information", "Supporting Evidence" or similar. In this box you should give your reasons for applying for the post and provide additional information to demonstrate how you match the person specification. This can include relevant skills, knowledge, experience, voluntary activities, training, etc. If you are applying for a research role, it is important to provide details about research experience, publications or poster presentations, clinical care (knowledge and skills) and clinical audit. You may or may not be restricted by word count, the space available may be expandable (i.e. NHS Jobs) and you might be told that you can "cut and paste" relevant sections from your CV. However, this is a statement, not a series of bullet points so it needs to be carefully constructed, like an essay, and should have an introduction, main body and conclusion. Again, do not forget to talk about your *accountability, professional standards and values* (NHS Employers 2014; NMC 2015a).

It helps to break down information into the following paragraph headings:

1. Reasons for applying and interest in the organisation
2. Recognition of the organisation's values and their alignment to your values
3. Specific area/s of interest
4. Placement experience
5. Personal skills
6. Further experience from the course
7. Reference to accountability, training and CPD
8. Personal interests
9. Final USPs (unique selling points)

Start with a strong and positive first sentence. Remember to indicate why you wish to work for this employer; this may be their excellent reputation or a new service initiative. With reference to point 3 above, some trusts will ring fence and advertise for a generic NQN/NQM Band 5 post rather than recruit for certain areas. Trusts that recruit early in the season to fill posts in 4–6 months' time may be unable to commit to vacancies being available within a speciality at the point at which you are ready to be employed. If you have a preference or wish to rank your preferences, you need to declare this within the personal statement and provide a clear rationale for the choice/s expressed.

You do not have to stick religiously to this order; you should write in a professional but personable style you feel comfortable with and use evidence of achievements to support statements. Again it is worth asking for professional advice about the content and sentiment. It is always wise to get a critical friend to proofread your work and spot those common errors (like "roll" and "role") that may go undetected through spellcheckers. Once you are confident it is ready, take a copy as you will need to refer back to this.

The employer will also be looking for examples of evidence-based practice (EBP) within the applicant's personal statement (supporting information). This is not just a case of putting in the odd reference against statements; approach this like an assignment and make sure that you refer to the most up-to-date evidence available, be it NICE guidance, DH policy or a review of best practice. This is also an opportunity to talk about the focus of your dissertation or a key assignment. Refer to the example in Box 3.24.

---

**BOX 3.24  An example of EBP in a personal statement**

"My interest in promoting breastfeeding to teenage mothers derived from reading an American study by Smith et al (2012) entitled 'Early Breastfeeding Experiences of Adolescent Mothers: A Qualitative Prospective Study'. This highlighted that a positive early breastfeeding experience and ongoing support systems increased a new mother's competency and thereby the likelihood of continuing the practice. During my last Year 2 placement I attended postnatal classes for teenage mothers and listened to individuals talking about how their feelings influenced their feeding practices. This was the catalyst for my final year dissertation which examined 'What kind of support, in the early days after an infant is born, is most likely to ensure that teenage mothers commit to and continue to breastfeed?' My findings have helped me to understand the impact of both formal and informal support systems and my role as a facilitator. I have been encouraged by my supervisor to submit a resumé for publication."

---

Two examples of personal statements are included in Boxes 3.25 and 3.26 to illustrate a variety of styles. The first was written by Sophie Jones and relates closely to her CV which you are already familiar with. The second one was written by Kate, a final year midwifery student; this secured her an interview which led ultimately to a job offer.

**BOX 3.25  A personal statement for Sophie Jones**

I am a student at the University of Southampton completing a Degree in Nursing (Adult). I decided to study nursing because I perceived it to be a vocation that is stimulating, varied, challenging, rewarding and ultimately fulfilling – my assumptions have proved to be correct. I am interested in medical nursing, particularly acute medical assessment and respiratory medicine, but also emergency medicine. The trust staff I have spoken to have inspired me with their commitment and enthusiasm. I know that X Trust has recently gained Foundation status and plans to increase its critical care facilities; it has an excellent reputation and I would be proud to work for such a progressive organisation.

Acute medicine is an area of nursing within which I can apply my full range of nursing skills. My Placement 5 (Autumn 2014) experience in the Acute Medical Unit at X Hospital, was one that I thrived in as I felt stretched mentally as well as physically. I became competent in admitting, assessing and prioritising the care of acutely unwell patients using NEWs and was confident enough to manage my own bay of four patients. This involved delegating to HCAs and junior students in my team. There was a fast turnover of patients and I am now also very adept at accepting and handing over patients and communicating concerns with the medical team. In my clinical assessment my mentor awarded me an "A" and commended me on my high standard of patient care and junior management skills. My drugs knowledge has grown substantially; I frequently acted as the second nurse checking medicines and am now familiar with e-prescribing.

My Placement 4 was with the community nursing team. I was privileged to be mentored by a highly skilled community matron and gained experience of how the virtual ward operates. I also worked for a week with the Rapid Response Team assessing patients whose conditions had deteriorated, considering ways in which admission could be avoided and a care package introduced in order to care for them at home. This demonstrated how critical it is to maintain good patient records and communicate well with the other teams/services involved and the role of in-reach and out-reach services to ensure that people with long-term conditions get the best care, with specialist input as necessary. Some patients I met on the respiratory ward (P3) were frequent users of acute and emergency services; gaining insight into how they can be effectively supported at home by the multi-disciplinary team widened my understanding of what is possible and how risk is managed. I also respect more the expertise that patients possess in terms of their conditions and ability to self-manage. My interest in how patient education can promote self-management skills stemmed from listening to a group of patients talking about their experiences of living with degenerative neurological conditions. This taught me to think more about nursing as a partner-ship, doing with, rather than doing to patients. Not all the people I met were elderly; there were a number of younger patients who lead very independent lives, suffice for routine health assessments or interventions such as dressings. My dissertation explores the lived patient experience and it's entitled "Can patient blogs help change the way we think at about patient care". This revealed a wealth of untapped information and I would like to share my findings by pub-lishing an article.

At the end of Year 2 students undertake a Personal Development Experience (PDE); this is a 3-week placement with learning outcomes that the student has to set up and negotiate. I chose to spend my time in the healthcare facility at HMP X in Devon. This is a Category C prison; many of the inmates have long-term health problems includ-ing mental health illness. It provided an insight into prison nursing, the assessment and treatment of primary and urgent unscheduled care needs from minor injuries to life-threatening emergencies such as hanging, substance misuse and associated mental health issues, predicting and managing aggression/violence and medicines man-agement in prisons. It made me revisit my values and beliefs and has made me more aware of the need to be open-minded, to listen carefully and to observe patients' non-verbal communication more closely.

The degree programme has encouraged me to be very organised and prioritise my workload. During P4 and P5 I had the opportunity to practise my teaching skills through presentations to my peers and junior students. When I started my course I was quite shy; now I can hold my own if I have to speak in public (i.e. handover, ward-rounds, case conferences or presentations) and feel confi-dent to challenge issues. The research skills I have learnt on the programme mean that if there is a question about any element of practice I can quickly search for an answer using the plethora of electronic database. For example, during my community place-ment I was introduced to silver impregnated dressings. It was being considered for a patient with a non-healing wound but there was concern about sensitivities. I offered to conduct a literature review and feedback to staff my findings before a change of prod-uct was agreed. The main discussion featured a document by the International Consensus (2012) – *Appropriate use of silver dressings in wounds. An expert working group consensus* (London: Wounds International). This was a very positive experience of evidence-based decision-making and made me realise how I can act as a role model, show initiative and take a lead in clinical practice.

I realise that as a registered nurse I am required to adhere to the Nursing and Midwifery Council's professional Code of Conduct (NMC

2015a) and to participate in life-long learning and continuing professional development. This will in part facilitate personal accountability and ensure that I comply with the trust's values (Solent NHS Trust 2014) and expectation that I am actively involved in clinical governance. I am a very motivated and self-directed learner who is aiming to achieve a first-class honours. Beyond this short-term goal, and looking ahead with enthusiasm to Placement 6 (June to August 2015), I will be focusing on further developing my junior leadership and management skills to be ready for my transition into a newly qualified nurse (NQN) Band 5 role in October 2015. This placement will be on the Cancer Care Unit in X Hospital. I have had some experience of caring for dying patients and their relatives but am keen to learn more about palliative care, in particular how to manage difficult conversations and promote dignified, person-centred care at the end of life. My other goal is to become more confident in assessing and effectively managing pain.

The ideal first NQN post would offer me the opportunity to progress clinically and academically through preceptorship, keeping up to date with mandatory skills training and undertaking further speciality-orientated study. I also chose this trust because it has established links with the university and invests in staff development. I would like to become a mentor to share my passion for nursing and support students. Long term I would be interested in undertaking Master's-level studies and potentially a nurse specialist role.

During term time and in addition to a busy study and placement programme, I do volunteer work twice a month with the Homeless Support Project in Southampton. This has opened my eyes to the needs of the homeless, particularly in relation to their health needs, their vulnerability and the stigma attached to being homeless. It has given me confidence to build relationships and deal with challenging situations such as an intoxicated client. At the university I am involved in the Student Union Fundraising Team; at Christmas I organised a "Bake Off" which raised £500 for UNICEF. My academic tutor put my name forward to be an ambassador for the faculty and this has proved to be a really rewarding experience. This involves giving talks to groups of college students who are interested in nursing as a career.

I am a keen football player, representing the university in the Women's 1st XI team and coordinating the fixtures list. In addition I enjoy open-water swimming, films and reading poetry as a means of relaxation. This balance enables me to cope with the demands of nursing. In patient testimonies I am described as "compassionate, approachable and extremely professional". I am able to say that I am a team player and someone who can be relied upon. I am wholly committed to making a difference to the patient's experience.

## BOX 3.26 Kate's personal statement for an NQM post

I am a keen and enthusiastic nearly-qualified midwife studying at the university. I am passionate about providing safe, effective care to women and their families throughout their journey to parenthood, as well as involving women in decisions regarding their care as much as they wish to be involved. I aim to normalise pregnancy and birth as far as possible for all women to give them the satisfaction they deserve. I am looking for a full-time position where I can consolidate my midwifery training and develop new skills in all areas of midwifery to help me become the autonomous practitioner I wish to be.

My placements have all been based in a regional unit for maternity and fetal medicine caring for a number of extremely high-risk mothers and babies. This has given me experience in some very complex cases ranging from placenta accreta to a variety of neonatal conditions and is something I wish to continue to be exposed to as a newly qualified midwife. The university and hospital are both heavily research based which has showed me the importance of evidence-based practice which I intend to continue throughout my career. During my time at university I have had placements in the community with both integrated and case-loading teams, on the labour ward and the alongside birthing centre, and on the high-risk antenatal and postnatal wards, as well as short placements on the neonatal unit, day assessment unit and an upcoming placement with the fetal medicine team. This variety of placements has given me experience in all areas of midwifery and has exposed me to the wonders and challenges of both high- and low-risk maternity care.

During my second year I carried out an elective placement with a sexual health service. This gave me an understanding of the management and treatment of sexually transmitted infections in and out of pregnancy. It also gave me insight into methods practitioners can use to disclose sensitive information in a compassionate and caring manner. The city has a very diverse population giving me experience caring for women from an array of socio-economic, cultural and religious backgrounds; and I have been involved in a number of safeguarding cases ranging from teenage pregnancy, domestic violence and drug abuse.

As part of my training I have been expected to carry out annual training updates in order to maintain competency and ensure safe practice – such as aseptic non-touch technique, basic life support and infection control. During my third year I have been working through the K2 CTG (cardiotocograms) analysis programme and attended a PROMPT (PRactical Obstetric Multi-Professional Training) study day, both of which highlighted the importance of multi-disciplinary working, good communication within a team, documentation and keeping up to date in regard to research, protocol and guidelines. I have also been a simulated patient for the PROMPT study day. Acting as the client helped me realise how important communication and debriefing with women and their partners is, especially during complex or emergency situations.

I am keen to continue learning throughout my career with an interest in gaining competency in cannulation, suturing and care for women with IV infusions and epidurals. I am particularly interested in completing the mentorship course as I am passionate about inspiring and educating the next generation of midwives. Throughout my time at university I have been involved with the faculty open days running drop in clinics about applications and skills sessions giving prospective students an insight to midwifery. Recently I also helped out at the midwifery selection day being involved on the panel for the group activity. Clinical audit is an integral part of clinical governance and service improvement. I have been involved in several audits throughout my training. One of these was an inter-professional learning project about nursing handovers in a neonatal unit and another regarding the role of the supervisor of midwives.

Throughout my training I have been commended on my thorough documentation; professional and confident manner with women, their families and other members of the multi-disciplinary team; and my knowledge base which underpins the care I provide, but also my willingness to ask for help and answers if I am uncertain of what to do. I pride myself on my punctuality, hardworking nature and perseverance when gaining new skills. I always work within the NMC Code of Conduct (2015) and follow guidelines and policy. I am a reflective practitioner and use my experiences – those that went well and those that did not – to help me develop and improve my practice.

I have good IT skills and use hospital computer systems such as HICCS and e-quest confidently. I also have a full driving licence and access to my own vehicle.

## HOW TO CREATE A PORTFOLIO FOR INTERVIEWS AND CPD

A portfolio serves as a dynamic record of achievement. Like your CV it will evolve with you as you progress through and beyond an education programme, gathering experience, knowledge and skills associated with your chosen discipline. Whilst not dissimilar to a school record of achievement, this portfolio focuses on your journey from a student into the role of an NQN/NQM and beyond, recording your CPD.

Once you are qualified you will be required to renew your registration through revalidation. To do this you must compile a portfolio which contains a minimum of five written reflections on the NMC Code (2015a) and a record of your CPD and practice-related feedback, as outlined in "How to revalidate with the NMC" (2015b). This document provides registrants with guidance and a series of templates to support the revalidation process. Furthermore, every registrant has to declare that they have complied with the revalidation requirements and may be asked to provide additional documentary evidence by means of a portfolio to verify the declaration.

During your undergraduate programme you can use the reflective accounts record log template (NMC 2015c, p. 5) or a similar agreed template to document additional evidence of practice development. This will also familiarise you with the format and get you in the habit of capturing and reflecting on experiences on the course that have had, and you anticipate will have, an impact on your future practice. The NMC template is provisional so please refer to the subsequent final guidance on their website.

For each placement, you should consider completing a minimum of two reflective accounts. On the NMC template are four questions:

1. What was the nature of the (CPD) activity/practice-related feedback?
2. What did you learn from the (CPD) activity and/or feedback?
3. How did you change or improve your work as a result?
4. How is this relevant to the Code?

The acronym in brackets (CPD) should be removed from the above wording as these reflections will be compiled from your perspective as a pre-registrant. When you write your personal statement these reflections will provide you with examples to illustrate; likewise in an interview you can select individual items to present to the panel. Coloured index flags/tabs help highlight key pages that you may wish to refer to to demonstrate a personal or professional quality or achievement. In addition, the portfolio is a good aide-memoire that you can read whilst waiting for the interview to remind you of all that you have accomplished on the course.

In terms of presentation, it is recommended you use a robust quality folder to house materials, placing individual items in plastic wallets. Include an index and order it in the same way you order your CV so that your most relevant achievement is at the front. Use dividers to break up sections into:

- CV at front – resumé
- Statement of academic integrity which confirms that the contents of the portfolio are authentic
- Personal statement/s
- Certificates mandatory updates (i.e. moving and handling; fire safety)
- Study days

- Modules (i.e. Open University; RCN online; RCM i-learn or university accredited)
- Educational achievements
- Awards or commendations
- Contributions to extra-curricular activities

Electronic assessment of practice portfolios (eFolio) offer enormous scope to include integrated tools such as a CV builder or a reference maker. This would give students the facility to transfer personal data and for placement information to be automatically copied into pre-formatted templates. The same would apply to final placement reports and the contact details of those who have agreed to supply a reference.

Here are links to four key resources that you will find helpful:

- Nursing and Midwifery Council (2015b) How to revalidate with the NMC – provisional guidance: requirements for renewing your registration and demonstrating your continuing fitness to practice. London: NMC (Online) www.nmc.org.uk/globalassets/sitedocuments/revalidation/how-to-revalidate-final-draft.pdf
- Nursing and Midwifery Council (2015c) NMC Templates. London: NMC (Online) www.nmc.org.uk/standards/revalidation/revalidation-guidance-and-resources/
- The RCN Learning Zone: this includes a CV builder and bite-sized modules for CPD www.rcn.org.uk/development/learning/learningzone
- The RCNi portfolio which is NMC compliant www.rcni.com/portfolio

## SUMMARY

The investment in this stage of the process will be enormous and should not be underestimated. This foundation work and the attention to detail should result in the offer of an interview. If it does not, then you need to know why and reflect on what you need to do in order to guarantee success next time. Never be afraid to ask for help.

# 4

# The Selection and Recruitment Process

## KEY WORDS

Job description; Agenda for Change; Knowledge and Skills Framework (KSF); NHS Constitution; Values-based recruitment; Minimum genuine occupational qualifications (GOQ); Screening; Shortlisting; Social networking and lifestyle; Selection; Requirements; Methods; Purpose of interviews; Types of interviews; Assessment centres; On-the-spot screening interviews; Assessment centres; Panel interviews; Classic one-to-one interviews; Multiple mini-interviews (MMIs); Telephone or webcam-based interviews; Presentations; Group interviews; Competency-based assessment; Role play and simulation; Numeracy and literacy assessments; Psychometric and aptitude tests; Equality Act; Discrimination

This section offers a unique insight into the employer's perspective in order for you to understand the process which underpins recruitment and selection. It will start by looking at how the formal pay and progression structure is used in conjunction with policy to create the job description. It will then examine values-based recruitment (VBR) and the emergent role of service users in recruitment processes. Consideration will be given to how employers will screen applications to produce a shortlist before reviewing the different ways of thereafter selecting the ideal candidate. The final section deals with the law pertaining to applications, interview conduct, disability and health and employment checks. There is also specific advice for overseas registrants wishing to work in the UK.

## THE JOB DESCRIPTION

The job description and associated salary must comply with specific requirements relating to pay and conditions and legislation. In the NHS pay scales are agreed nationally on an annual basis. An independent healthcare provider can choose to mirror the public sector pay scale, with or without additional employee benefits. Understanding how pay and pay progression are determined is an important part of your transition into qualified employment and beyond. Agenda for Change (AfC) (DH 2004) was introduced to provide a clear definition of the level of knowledge and skills required for each post. It modernised the pay and conditions for both nurses and midwives. A newly qualified practitioner will enter at Band 5 and there will be an outline set of competencies, known as the Knowledge and Skills Framework (KSF), for this role. There are six core dimensions present in every job outline (Box 4.1) and then 2–6 specific dimensions taken from a comprehensive list of 24. Within each dimension there are four levels; the higher the level, the higher the level of skill and knowledge required to fulfil the post (RCN 2014b).

---

**BOX 4.1 The six core dimensions of Agenda for Change (DH 2004)**

1. Communication
2. Personal and people development
3. Health, safety and security
4. Service improvement
5. Quality
6. Equality and diversity

---

In the most recent review of AfC (NHS Staff Council 2013) there were two key changes that affect all staff. These are:

- Progression through all incremental pay points in all pay bands to be conditional on individuals demonstrating that they meet locally agreed performance requirements in line with Annex W (England) of the AfC handbook.
- The removal of accelerated pay progression associated with preceptorship for staff joining pay band 5 as new entrants.

However, it is the second change that has the most significant impact on graduates moving into employment, both within and outside the NHS, as it removed the remuneration associated with the completion of preceptorship. Currently Band 5 starts at £21,478 and has eight progression points taking it to a maximum of £27,901. With additional postgraduate qualifications a newly qualified health visitor will commence on Band 6 (£25,783 to £34,530) (RCN 2014c). To facilitate a working understanding of the KSF there are a number of useful short guidance booklets (RCN 2006, 2007a, 2009) available on the RCN website, which should be read in conjunction with the NHS KSF handbook (NHS Staff Council 2014a, 2014b). The most up-to-date pay scales can be found on the NHS Careers website. When you look more closely at salaries you will see some variation by location. Historically referred to as "weightings", supplements can be added to the basic rate of pay for jobs in Inner London, Outer London and Fringe locations.

The supplement compensates for the higher cost of living so for Inner London this equates to 20 per cent of basic salary (minimum payment of £4,076 up to a maximum of £6,279 (RCN 2014c; NHS Careers 2014)). Any salary uplift should be factored into your cost/benefit analysis if you are looking at jobs in areas where the cost of living (rent, council tax, public transport, etc.) is above that of the national average.

## ESSENTIAL SKILLS

The employer will use the KSF framework competencies to compile the job description. There will be little variation in a generic Band 5 profile; however, look carefully for currency. Trusts will annually review and revise roles as necessary; if they have reviewed but not made any changes, then this should be clear by the date on the document. They will also produce a person specification which stipulates the genuine minimum requirement and genuine occupational qualifications (GOQ) required in order to effectively perform the job. Applicants must have current UK professional registration or, in the case of those applying whilst still being students, they must be on a programme that leads to professional registration.

The job description and person specification will help you complete your application so you need to download copies. Print off two copies of each – one for reference only and to take to interview, and a second one which you will use as a working document and make notes on.

Now complete Activity 4.1.

### ACTIVITY 4.1

**The key components of a Band 5 job description**

You will need a copy of a Band 5 job description:

- Enrol on NHS Jobs (if not already enrolled).
- Search for a Band 5 job by discipline (nurse or midwife) and field.
- Narrow your search by specialism.
- Narrow by location.
- Select a job that appeals to you and print off the advert.
- Print off the documents attached to the advert (you will refer to these later).
- Locate the organisation's values (usually within the advert or on their website).

- Read the job description:
  - Highlight the key competencies.
  - Tick those that you can demonstrate evidence of achievement.
- Read the person specification:
  - Look at the prerequisites and desirable skills and tick those you can provide.

## VALUES-BASED RECRUITMENT

Both the Francis report's findings (Mid Staffordshire NHS Foundation Trust Public Inquiry 2013) and the Kirkup (2015) report into maternity and neonatal services at the University Hospitals of Morecambe Bay NHS Foundation Trust have added fuel to rising concerns about care standards, serious failings and the attitudes and behaviour of health-care professionals. The question is how can we be sure we are recruiting the right people with the right skills and values? All students and registrants need to adhere to the standards set out in the revised Code (NMC 2015a). Divided into four sections (**P**rioritising people; **P**ractise effectively; **P**reserve safety; **P**romote professionalism and trust), the message is very clear – "While you can interpret the values and principles set out in the Code in a range of different practice settings, they are not negotiable or discretionary".

Values-based recruitment (VBR) is an approach that helps organisations to recruit individuals who are most closely aligned with the values of an organisation (The Health Foundation 2014). It is used to screen applicants for nursing and midwifery programmes (Miller and Bird 2014). In the case of the NHS it is about selecting and recruiting applicants whose values and behaviours are most closely aligned with those set out in the NHS Constitution (DH 2013b). In order to be reliable, VBR practices should be "equality assessed and assured" (NHS Employers 2014).

Specific values are set out in a number of key documents that govern your profession and, more widely, employing organisations. Without exception every undergraduate should have a sound theoretical and practical understanding of the 6Cs of nursing (care, compassion, competence, communication, courage and commitment) (DH 2012). These relate to the fundamental principles of professional practice and there is an expectation that you will be able to provide evidence at interview to show how these are embedded in your practice. At service level the overarching values which under-pin the NHS in England are clearly set out in the NHS Constitution (DH 2013b). Founded on seven key principles and values (Box 4.2), the Constitution applies to all staff, in both clinical and non-clinical NHS roles, including local authority public health services and their employers. Moreover it includes staff wherever they are employed, whether in public, private or voluntary sector organisations that pro-vide services to the NHS (DH 2013b).

---

**BOX 4.2 The NHS Constitution's seven key principles (DH 2013b)**

1. The NHS provides a comprehensive service, available to all.
2. Access to NHS services is based on clinical need, not an individual's ability to pay.
3. The NHS aspires to the highest standards of excellence and professionalism.
4. The NHS aspires to put patients at the heart of everything it does.
5. The NHS works across organisational boundaries and in partnership with other organisations in the interest of patients, local communi-ties and the wider population.
6. The NHS is committed to providing best value for taxpayers' money and the most effective, fair and sustainable use of finite resources.
7. The NHS is accountable to the public, communities and patients that it serves.

---

Graduating students are expected to promote and uphold these seven core principles and values. In addition, the organisation (i.e. trust) you would like to work for has almost certainly published its own set of values derived from those of the NHS. Box 4.3 contains an example of how one trust's values are encapsulated in the acronym "INSPIRE" (Solent NHS Trust 2014). Again, you need to acknowledge the importance of both sets (NHS and trust) and make explicit refer-ence to them in accompanying personal statements and at interview. The employer may also test your values through other means such as pre-screening assessments, role play and written responses to sce-narios (Miller 2015). These are the benchmarks by which the trust is judged, so prospective employees will be expected to know what the values are and show a commitment to upholding them. Furthermore, it has been proposed that registered staff appraisals use a values-based framework to assess CPD needs (DH 2013c).

## BOX 4.3 An example of one trust's values

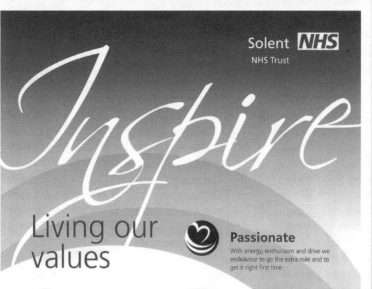

Solent **NHS**
NHS Trust

# Living our values

 **Passionate**
With energy, enthusiasm and drive we endeavour to go the extra mile and to get it right first time.

 **Involved**
We strive to involve, engage and value individuals, teams and patients.

 **Innovative**
We are creating the future through researching new and improved ways of working and adopting best practice.

 **Nurturing Talent**
We are committed to providing a learning environment that nurtures talent and achieves successful outcomes.

 **Respectful**
We are respectful of individuals, services and organisations, by being transparent and honest and our actions reflect our words through our integrity.

 **Striving for excellence**
We are proud about the quality of our work and continually strive to exceed expectations for patients and staff.

**Empowered**
We are all empowered to participate, communicate, innovate and lead by being accountable and responsible for everything we do.

Our values guide our everyday actions and ensure that we are all working towards a shared goal of providing the highest quality care to our patients. We are proud to have developed the above values which have been adopted as the acronym "INSPIRE".

Reproduced with permission from Solent NHS Trust (2014)

## SERVICE-USER INVOLVEMENT IN RECRUITMENT AND SELECTION

In addition to the NHS Mandate to recruit for values in the NHS, organisations are beginning to actively look at how they can increase public and patient involvement (PPI) in the selection and recruitment of staff at all levels from undergraduate to qualified positions. This is in response to key drivers such as recommendations for "Transforming participation in health care" (NHS England 2013), the concept of "People Powered Health" and the view that "the NHS belongs to us all". Representatives of users and carers bring their unique views about treatment and care, can help set priorities and challenge outmoded assumptions (NHS Wales 2010). PPI is not exclusive to the NHS; there are best practice examples of universities, county councils, charities and voluntary sector harnessing the expertise of reference groups including children and young people (Gloucestershire County Council 2005; Teeside University 2014; Participation Works 2015).

Employers should be engaging with service users and carers at the start of the process in the design or review of job descriptions, person specifications and advertisements and then later on in the shortlisting and interviewing of applicants. Graduates therefore need to anticipate the possibility that applications may be scrutinised by appropriately trained service users working in partnership with the employer. They may also be setting questions and there in person at the interview itself. You can find examples of questions set by service users later on in this chapter in section "Numeracy and Literacy Assessment" and Chapter 5. In Box 4.4 is an account provided by one user of mental health services and another by a carer who sits on the trust interview panels. This clearly identifies what is expected.

---

**BOX 4.4 Service users' reflections about being part of an interview panel**

**Louise**: *"I have sat on several interview panels recruiting CAMHS professionals. The main thing I look at is how the interviewee interacts with me. This gives an indication of how they would relate to service users. I look for someone who is treating me as an equal, interacting with me as they do the other panellists, making eye contact, smiling, shaking my hand. Ideally the interviewees would adapt their answers so as a service user I can understand them; however, there is a fine balance between this and being patronising, explaining every obvious detail."*

**Brian**: *"I feel that meeting service users and carers is extremely important as these are the people they will be involved with once qualified. I feel we also provide a unique perspective in terms of evaluating their communication skills, confidence in dealing with others and their ability to make us feel comfortable and at ease in their presence."*

## THE VALUE-ADDED ELEMENT

The applicant may also have other experiences and skills that an employer is interested in understanding and capitalising on. The proverb "all work and no play makes Jack a dull boy" means that outside interests prevent boredom and the risk of being one dimensional. People with interesting backgrounds and hobbies will stand out; an interviewer admitted that if the candidate is soulless and boring it makes for a very short interview! There is significant value in public recognition, so if you have had an award or commendation at school, college or university or for community achievements, then you need to draw attention to this. University life provides students with the chance to represent the student's voice in faculty activities such as open days, undergraduate selection days, and student and staff committees. Engagement in sports clubs and societies or volunteering with external youth organisations or community projects (e.g. Scouts, St John Ambulance, Duke of Edinburgh's Award scheme and sports coaching) paints a picture of someone who is actively contributing to the wider society. Many students will be working for healthcare agencies, trust banks or part-time in other jobs; appreciating that there are undoubtedly financial reasons for this, this experience also needs to be described in such a way as to make it relevant and attractive to the employer.

## THE IDEAL CANDIDATE

So how do recruiters identify who they want to interview? This question was posed to two local recruiters, one NHS based, one a private employer. A summary of their answers is in Box 4.5.

### BOX 4.5 Screening – the employer's perspective

- How do you identify from a pile of applications which applicants you will invite to interview? Answer: *Those who*
  - *Possess the minimum genuine occupational requirements and qualifications (GORs/GOQs) and pass screening criteria*
  - *Express an explicit interest in working for us*

- *Have experience in a specialism but it is not essential for NQN/Ms*
- *Have paid attention to detail (presentation, formality, spelling, grammar and punctuation)*
- What else can applicants do to make sure they get through this crucial part of the selection process? Answer: *Those who*
  - *Show passion for your occupation and career choices*
  - *Talk about values and the 6Cs (DH 2012, 2013b)*
  - *Bring fresh thinking and ideas into discussions*
  - *Incorporate examples of evidence-based practice (EBP)*
  - *Talk about prior experience or interest in specialism (may not always have had placement experience but could be agency, visits or subject of dissertation that shows this)*
  - *Demonstrate engagement in extra-curricular activities (university societies, community, voluntary or charitable work in UK or abroad)*
  - *Identify personal successes, that is, student of the year, outstanding achievements or marks*
- If you reject an application, can the person contact you to discuss why? What advice would you give them? Answer:
  - *Candidates will need to contact us for this. We do not give written feedback, but we will give outline verbal feedback.*

## SCREENING APPLICATIONS

Essentially the recruiter will use the list of required and desirable characteristics in the person specification to screen applications. Some advertisements will stipulate that the post is only for newly qualified staff; if it is a generic Band 5 and there are no restrictions then this is open to all. The selector will be looking to see that the applicant has tailored the contents to the job. A selector may use designated software to help them sift through applications to see how often all key words from the job advertisement appear in the job application. If you are submitting a number of applications for different jobs make sure that you amend the contents accordingly. Under pressure it is easy to make a costly mistake. You do not want to be rejected because you have got the name of the employing trust, department or service wrong.

Often qualifying students are hesitant about competing with experienced staff and deterred by the phrase "experience is desirable". They may also have been given out-of-date advice, like Ian (Box 4.6). "Experience desirable" in fact means experience is not a necessity and the organisation would consider appointing a newly qualified practitioner who shows potential and would fit into the team.

> **BOX 4.6 Ian's story**
>
> *"I qualified in 2008 and immediately applied as a community psychiatric nurse within Older Persons Mental Health. In nursing the written rule was that 'You had to spend at least two years on a ward before applying into the community' but I spoke with the manager of the service, explained my previous skills and qualifications (in social care) and was told to apply.*
>
> *I was offered the job as a Band 5. In my third month other nurses said they felt newly qualified nurses should not be in my position. So using some of the skills taught to me at university (presentation and research) I took the opportunity and spoke at two nursing conferences justifying why newly qualified nurses were able to take on community roles. This seemed to take hold and very soon other newly qualified nurses were getting community positions."*

To ensure that the screening process is fairly conducted, there will be a screening checklist, to ensure that the applicant:

- Has the minimum GOQs or is applying for registration within a defined timescale
- Completed all parts of the application
- Provided the required numbers of referees
- Included a supporting statement
- Talks about the trust/department by name
- Refers to their professional **ACCOUNTABILITY** (NMC 2015a)
- Includes examples of **EBP**
- Paid attention to detail and there is evidence of proofreading

It is usual to score each element of the application; if essential elements are missing then the application will be rejected. Some sections within electronic applications are mandatory so if you do not put information in a section, it will automatically stop you from submitting, highlight what is missing and let you correct it before proceeding to the next step. However, it is accuracy in every section that counts and the quality of the content in any "free text" section.

## SOCIAL NETWORKING AND LIFESTYLE

The Internet provides easy access to social networking sites such as LinkedIn, Facebook and Twitter. These sites are an integral part of many people's lives. Arguably an individual's "social media identity" is not created for the purposes of securing a job (Kwoh 2012). On this premise companies would have difficulty defending a rejection if they illegally used information (for example about race or gender); however, evidence of disloyalty, dishonesty or behaviours that would bring the profession into disrepute would raise concerns and bias decisions. Whilst it is good practice to ask permission, do not assume that any employer or recruitment agency who wants to perform additional background checks on you, will do so. If someone had good reason to conduct a background search for additional information on you, then what would they find? If you are not sure, then "Google yourself". Ask yourself, "Would I employ this person on the basis of what I see?" Think about whether or not the information portrays the key professional credentials that match the type of employer values in Box 4.3. If there is information in the public domain such as affiliation to political groups, that may potentially harm your job prospects, you need to manage your profile and should either restrict access or better still remove it entirely. Indiscrete remarks and breaches of confidentiality are fitness for practice issues (NMC 2012a, 2015a).

So in summary, the screening process forms a key part of reducing down the applicant pool to those who are, on paper, potentially best suited to the job. It therefore really pays to clean up your online image, removing any unsuitable photos or messages. The same applies to voicemail out of office recordings. First impressions count.

## TYPES OF SELECTION METHODS

Employers use a variety of tried and tested methods to identify their ideal candidate. A major part of your preparation will need to be based around the style of interview of which there are a number of approaches:

1. "On the spot" screening interviews
2. Assessment centres
3. Panel interviews
4. Classic one-to-one interviews
5. Multiple mini-interviews (MMIs)
6. Telephone or webcam based
7. Presentations
8. Group interviews
9. Competency-based assessment (includes role play and simulation)
10. Numeracy and literacy assessments
11. Psychometric and aptitude tests

Before looking at the specifics of each of the above, it is important to consider what the purpose of an interview is. There are two perspectives: that of the candidate and that of the interviewer. Interviewees will be looking to use the opportunity to:

- Be treated equitably
- Demonstrate their suitability for the job
- Effectively communicate key information about themselves, their motivation and keenness to work for the employer
- Demonstrate attributes that they may find difficult to convey on paper applications
- Ask questions of the employer about the organisation and the job
- Help them decide whether or not this is an employer they would wish to work for, if offered a job

In contrast, this is when the interviewer will:

- Have the chance to communicate face to face with a prospective employee
- Assess the candidate's preparation for interview and importantly suitability for the role
- Evaluate communication skills, self-awareness, attitudes and knowledge base
- Pose questions that test a candidate's responses to practical scenarios and professional accountability
- Ask more probing questions and seek clarification over uncertainties
- Judge the candidate's motivation, perceived level of commitment and long-term potential
- Imagine the individual in role, as a member of a team or leading a team caring for patients, engaging with visitors and other professionals
- Check qualifications and essential documentation such as registration and visas
- Select the strongest candidate
- Choose not to employ an individual

Interviewing is very resource-intensive and costly so some organisations may outsource this activity to a specialist healthcare agency who will recruit on their behalf. This is often how overseas recruitment for UK trusts is organised. If you are applying from outside of the UK you may be invited to attend large selection events in your own country, in venues such as a hotel or conference facility. The same applies to overseas recruiters, for example, working on behalf of the Canadian or Australian government health departments, who travel to the UK and Eire to recruit UK midwives and nurses for target areas such as obstetrics, paediatrics, intensive care or theatres.

## THE "ON THE SPOT" SCREENING INTERVIEW

Sometimes employers will offer "on the spot" interviews; this might be during an informal visit to an organisation, a formal open day held by the employer (e.g. a trust open day), an event recruiting staff for overseas employment (i.e. for a Middle East hospital) or at a careers fair. There may be a quiet area assigned for one-to-one meetings. If invited, you have of course the right to decline; however, if you have prepared for this possibility, you may well feel this is one opportunity not to be missed. Organisations may use this as a form of screening; if they do not feel that you are well placed to apply, then this is their opportunity to advise you accordingly and suggest how to gain extra qualifications or experience prior to applying at a later date. Conversely this may be the point at which you are encouraged to apply for a formal interview or even possibly offered a job there and then. If you anticipate an "on the spot interview" and want to proceed, do make sure you take all the necessary documentation with you (refer to Chapter 5, section "Documentation").

## ASSESSMENT CENTRES

An "assessment centre" is the term used to describe a recruitment event staged by an employer usually on their own premises. It is less often a designated building used solely for the purposes of assessment (Innes 2012b). Viewed as an advance on interview-only approaches to selection, they have grown in popularity since the 1950s when they were introduced primarily to improve the quality of military recruitment (Maldé 2007). This format continues to be used by the armed forces and police, large trusts and organisations such as local authorities recruiting new staff in volume at a given point, rather than for sporadic single posts.

During the assessment centre experience, candidates may be interviewed using just one or a combination of techniques such as one-to-one interviews, a drug assessment exercise, critical incident activities, group interviews, aptitude and psychometric tests. This triangulation can give a more robust picture of an individual's capabilities, hence its adoption by public services such as the NHS. Candidates need to be well prepared for this mixed method approach and encouraged to treat this as a positive learning experience (Maldé 2007). It is a time-intensive experience (that may last all day) and concentration is key; it will be hard work, stressful and tiring for any candidate. This link http://targetjobs.co.uk/careers-advice/assessment-centres gives more detail on individual components, but it is not specifically for nursing and midwifery graduates. The following sections look more closely at the different techniques.

## PANEL INTERVIEWS

This is one of the more traditional formats and the one that is most familiar to graduates with prior interview experience. The panel will comprise two or more people; this is in line with good interview practice guidance (Southern Health NHS Foundation Trust 2014). At least one of the panel members should have attended a recruitment and selection training course and will have considerable experience in conducting interviews. One person will chair the interview, managing the allocated time and who asks which question. Another will be taking notes but try not to be distracted by this. For NQN/M (generic Band 5) appointments one can expect panel members to be drawn from across a range of services, not just the areas that you have expressed an interested in. This will include senior clinical staff and department managers with representation from human resources and potentially a service user. Please refer to section "Types of Selection Methods" that talks specifi-cally about public and patient involvement in staff selection. Do not assume that the most experienced interviewer is the chair; this role may be rotated to offer less-experienced staff practice. Furthermore, you may be introduced to junior staff who will be observing for their own development; they may be asked to contribute so should not be disregarded during discussions. The skill you need to rehearse is to be able to communicate effectively, verbally and non-verbally with all members of the panel.

## ONE-TO-ONE INTERVIEWS

This may well be the choice for the smaller employer or indeed an individual (such as a service user) recruiting qualified staff as personal assistants. Inevitably the decision to employ rests on the subjective judgement of one person. It is tempting for applicants to try to win friends by taking a more relaxed stance and using humour (Innes 2012b). The rapport should remain professional at all times; there will be plenty of time to get to know your employer when you are working for them.

## MULTIPLE MINI-INTERVIEWS (MMIS)

MMIs are increasingly part of nursing and midwifery undergraduate applicant selection, so it may be that you have recent experience of this "speed-dating" style of format where you had to rotate through a series of 5–10 interview stations, each with a different examiner (Eva et al 2004; Young-Powell 2013). At each station there would have been a short, timed practical activity or question to answer. At undergraduate level the activities are usually quite generic, for example, "*Tell me, what do you see in this picture?*"; a role play with "*an upset classmate*" or a question such as "*Should alcoholics get liver transplants?*", the aim being to assess how candidates communicate and make decisions and ethical judgements.

If, however, applicants have to demonstrate a specific level of clinical expertise (such as at postgraduate level) a series of objective structured clinical examinations (OSCEs) based on clinical scenarios is a more appropriate format. Alongside the MMIs or OSCE there will also be traditional interview questions. It is argued that this multiple sampling approach based on a more practical assessment of what candidates are capable of doing allows greater insight into candidate abilities, thereby reducing interviewer bias.

Universities (i.e. Leeds, UEA and Birmingham) who use MMIs will often give examples on their websites so that students can prepare themselves for this type of interview. There is a plethora of discipline-specific resources including the bestselling book by Picard and Lee (2013).

## TELEPHONE OR VIDEO INTERVIEWS

Interviews do not have to be conducted face to face. Telephone interviews are more convenient, expedient and less resource-intensive so they tend to be used in the first instance to shortlist or for first interviews. This is then followed up with a face-to-face interview or assessment. Conference call facilities mean that there may be more than one person conducting the telephone interview. Personnel do not have to be co-located, that is, in the same office or on the same site. This is useful when recruiters and candidates are at a distance plus there are cost savings with respect to travel and accommodation. Arguably, since no one can be seen, dress code and body language become irrelevant. Yet as much, if not more, skill is required on the part of the interviewee to come over well. Some roles may require a lot of telephone communication (i.e. triage, advice lines or counselling services) so the employer may see this as an ideal way to ascertain how well the applicant can work remotely with this medium. Common courtesies are essential and there is more emphasis on the intonation of replies and subtleties heard within the message. One advantage is that the candidate can have notes in front of them that the recruiter cannot see.

Stepping beyond the relatively simple telephone interview, more organisations are considering and investing in the use of mobile technology, such as Skype, as an interview method. This can help manage and pre-screen a large volume of applicants. Advancements may soon include 3D video call technology. Webcams can literally and visually screen candidates to gain an early first impression and evaluate applicants for jobs. Again the interview panel do not need to all be in the same location.

This method relies heavily on computer and communication skills and therefore this is a distinct disadvantage to those who are less computer-literate or camera-shy. It is very difficult to demonstrate effective communication skills and convey confidence when you are so preoccupied with concerns about the technology working. Both parties should have an expert around to assist should problems occur with the transmission (dropped calls or disruption). In addition, the risk of someone else picking up the call, unexpected interruptions (such as people coming into the room unannounced, the phone ringing or a dog barking), needs to be managed and any background noise eliminated. Box 4.7 provides some top tips for webcam interview candidates.

---

**BOX 4.7 Top tips for webcam interviews**

1. Technology
   - *Rehearse with a friend on Skype so you feel comfortable.*
   - *Check the Internet connection, sound and image quality.*
2. Environment
   - *Choose a quiet room.*
   - *Turn off mobile phones/telephones off the hook.*
   - *Avoid rooms with an echo.*
   - *Position the computer in a well-lit area.*
   - *Avoid a plain white background.*
   - *Choose a background that looks business-like and tidy.*
3. Body language
   - *Turn body to corner and rotate head to screen looking into webcam.*
   - *Avoid looking at your own image.*

- *Pay attention to eye contact.*
- *Look pleased to meet the interviewer who may also be new to web interviews.*
- *Convey warmth and confidence in your responses.*
4. Dress
   - *Professional as you would for an interview, that is, suit/jacket.*
   - *Brighter solid colours are good if you have a pale complexion.*
   - *Avoid bold prints – opt instead for subdued prints.*
   - *Apply a little more make-up than usual.*
   - *Use a mirror to check final appearance before you go "live".*

The better candidates are those who have rehearsed with the technology and critically reviewed their performance (Williams 2013). Most careers services should offer this impartial and confidential facility. Web interviews are easy to record for training purposes and help people to see the messages that they may unconsciously send one another. The interaction, like face-to-face interviews, is still a very intense experience, but it does not go outside the confines of the "chat room". This is a major downside of Skype (Kiviat 2009). Candidates do not have an opportunity to get a true feel for the environment. Photographs can be deceptive and they may only show those specific elements of the venue that the employer wishes to share. There is no chance to explore a locality in person nor can they meet the wider staff and patients. How many people buy a holiday based on the glossy pictures in a brochure only to be disappointed when they arrive and find the resort half-built? If it is not possible to visit in advance, Google Earth is one way to take an independent virtual tour ahead of the interview.

If you are advised that the interview will be via Skype, then it is recommended that you watch this short 5-minute video by Kiviat (2010), which can be accessed via http://content.time.com/time/video/player/0,32068,46937715001_1933401,00.html.

## PRESENTATIONS

Pre-qualification nursing and midwifery assessments often require students to give presentations to their peer group, so this should not be a totally new experience. The recruiter may give all applicants the same topic or a range of topics to select from and should provide a laptop and projection facilities. They will be looking for evidence of organisation, preparation and rehearsal, in addition to how you structure content and your ability to communicate effectively, both verbal and through a visual medium such as PowerPoint or Prezi. Attention to detail and timings are essential; the audience will be expecting a high-quality performance and fresh thinking. Imagery and the use of cue cards can help dampen nerves. There is always the temptation to read aloud a scripted presentation but this can result in a very stilted and stiff delivery. It is really important to keep to the time allocated; if you overrun the interviewer can ask you to stop.

This format allows students the opportunity to demonstrate their strengths in terms of presentation skills, breadth and depth of evidence-based knowledge and practice application. In the conclusion, time should be allocated for audience questions and to thank them for listening. It is good practice to give each panel member a top-quality printed copy of the presentation so that they can refer back to this.

## GROUP INTERVIEWS

This format is used in the selection of undergraduate nurses and midwives so some students may have experience of this. It is less frequently used in the recruitment of NQN/Ms. However, this scenario enables employers to assess how individuals might work within a team setting. The set group activity could be either verbal or physical, that is, role play. Instinctively individuals will take one of a variety of roles (Belbin Associates 2011) as summarised in Table 4.1. Organisations will be looking to identify certain strengths and allowable weakness, whilst at the same time avoiding employing those who demonstrate poor self-awareness or negative traits that will not complement those within an existing team. For example the person who dominates discussions and shows an inability to accommodate or respect the views of others. And conversely the quiet individual who no one noticed.

Whilst applicants may be competing against one another for the prize of a job, they should not view each other as the enemy (Innes 2012b). The selector/s will be carefully watching applicants from the moment they meet; the task is important to give purpose to the group, but it is the nature and quality of social interactions before, during and after an activity that the observer/s will focus on. They will be interested in where the applicant positions themselves within the group, whether they initiate introductions and cooperate.

| TABLE 4.1 Belbin's 9 Team Role Descriptions (Belbin Associates 2011) | | |
|---|---|---|
| Plants | Coordinators | Team workers |
| Resource | Implements | Shapers |
| Monitor | Completers | Specialist |

Source: www.belbin.com/content/page/49/BELBIN(uk)-2011-TeamRoleSummary Descriptions.pdf

Do they appear to have understood the remit and importantly, what is this individual's role in achieving the desired outcome? Does the person demonstrate independence of thought and originality in their contributions and can they give and receive constructive criticism? Recruiters will use the scenario to help them get a feel for an individual's attitudes and values and how they might interact in practice, with patients, parents, relatives and other professionals in the multi-disciplinary team. In essence, is this person a team player, someone who listens and responds with professionalism?

A good performance must be sustained right up until the last minute. In some instances the programme may include refreshment breaks and lunch. Inevitably a few people will inadvertently drop their guard and this may adversely influence the outcome. At the end of a group interview, one candidate started talking to another about themselves, in effect speaking over the recruiter. As a result they missed essential instruction about what they would be doing next so looked foolish because they had to ask for the instruction to be repeated. Furthermore whilst others politely acknowledged the selector as they left the room, this candidate continued with their private conversation, totally ignoring the selector. After creating an initial good impression during the task, their exit showed a lack of respect and common courtesies.

## COMPETENCY-BASED ASSESSMENT

This section will look at two forms of competency-based assessment:

- Competency-based questioning
- Role play and simulated practice

All nursing and midwifery students experience competency-based assessment during clinical practice. However, taking this concept into an alien interview setting generates an understandable level of anxiety. If you are not yet competent in practice, then you will have the opportunity to try again; competency-based interviews are less forgiving as there is just one chance to prove yourself. The job description should clearly establish the level of competency – or capability – required to fulfil a defined role. Whilst the pre-registration preparation will have defined levels of competency at each progression point (i.e. end of Year 1, end of Year 2, upon qualification) and indicate achievement, employers may want to independently test out an individual's capability either by questioning them in a face-to-face interview or using an assessed activity such as role play or simulated practice. Both look at how a candidate approaches a specific task or situation, drawing on their skills and experiences. Look at the following examples of competency-based questions in Box 4.8 and think about how you might answer them.

---

**BOX 4.8 Examples of competency-based questions**

- What techniques do you use to prioritise your workload?
- How did you cope with a difficult situation that arose in practice?
- Can you give me an example of when you have helped a client to successfully overcome a barrier to regaining health?

---

Each question is asking for a brief story outlining the situation, justifying your actions and importantly demonstrating the value of your actions. Chapter 5, section "How to Construct a Good Answer" examines how to structure an effective answer using the Context, Action, Result (CAR) technique.

In the simulated practice scenario applicants will be expected to actively adopt the role of the nurse or midwife. All students will have undergone basic life support training and be familiar with skills rooms and CPR manikins; some scenarios will involve applicants demonstrating their response to an emergency situation, for example, *"Imagine you find a collapsed patient; they are not breathing. Demonstrate how you would approach this situation."*

Recent undergraduates may also be familiar with more sophisticated and interactive patient simulator technology such as SimMan, SimMom and SimBaby (Laerdal®). This computer-controlled facility can test a variety of attributes and knowledge, including how well candidates communicate whilst at the same time demonstrating mastery of defined practical nursing or midwifery skills. These might include management of the post-operative patient, a client having a seizure, a child in respiratory distress or an obstetric emergency. Those students with prior experience of simulated practice will remember how quickly they "slip" into role, behaving as if the dummy is human. They might be assessed individually or as part of a team of candidates who have been assigned to care for a patient (Box 4.9).

---

**BOX 4.9 An example of a mental health scenario**

Ed has just been sectioned under Section 3 of the Mental Health Act and has arrived on the unit. You have been asked by the nurse in charge to admit him and ensure that Ed understands what Section 3 means:

- During the admission Ed will indicate he is at high risk of self-harm.
- You will be expected to demonstrate how you will deal with this.

When appropriate organisations can employ real people, who may be service users or actors to play out the scripted role of a patient, relative or member of staff, the candidate must then respond as they would in practice. This is a good way of testing out personal attributes such as compassion and empathy, for example, when dealing with an anxious or depressed client. The characters will have been briefed to respond naturally to the candidate and should not deviate from the story or attempt to trip up the candidate. The very human nature of the interaction helps even the most self-conscious or tongue-tied person ease into the role.

Recording candidates allows recruiters more time to replay and examine the detail before making a final decision. Candidates should always have been pre-warned and consent to being filmed.

## NUMERACY AND LITERACY ASSESSMENT

The assessment of practice and theoretical assessment contained within undergraduate programmes tests students' proficiency in maths and English. Employers know that students very often have outside help compiling their application forms and personal statements. Therefore some will insist on independently appraising a candidate's numeracy and literacy as part of the pre-employment screening, thereby to ensure that all employees have a minimum agreed level in order to practise safely. The tests will be set under exam conditions; candidates will be told whether or not calculators are permitted. Any request for extra time must be submitted in advance (i.e. for those applicants who have dyslexia or need special adjustments for other reasons).

Overseas applicants will be required to demonstrate proficiency in comprehension, written and verbal English through successful attainment of the International English Language Testing System (IELTS) exam. The required level for nursing and midwifery is currently set at 7.0 (Glasper 2013). Furthermore foreign applicants will usually have to complete the overseas nursing programme (ONP) lasting 3–6 months. This is designed to ensure that they are equally as competent as any UK registrant. This includes a working knowledge of UK terminology (e.g. a stretcher is called a gurney in the US). For more information visit www.ielts.org.

Some organisations are now asking external partner agencies (i.e. patient groups or charities) or co-opted service users to set short answer questions that delve into the applicant's values, beliefs and attitudes whilst at the same time looking for clarity about their professional accountability. These may be marked externally and the feedback used in the decision-making process. An example might be:

- What is more important to you – paperwork or my care? Write your answer in no more than 250 words.

Assessment of numeracy skills can take place in many different formats ranging from short answer questions in a formal exam to problem-solving incorporated within a role-play scenario, for example:

- *Working out total urine output for 24 hours by adding up hourly recorded volumes*
- *Converting a newborn's weight from kgs to pounds and ounces*
- *Working out time lapse from point when casualty was found (07:47) and arrival of assistance (08:15)*

In addition, numeracy skills are tightly aligned with competent and safe medicines management. Given this is a key responsibility of all qualified nurses and midwives, it is reasonable to expect there will be an element of the assessment that relates to this. This may be in the form of a drug calculations exam. In preparation it is recommended that you access the resources in Box 4.10:

---

**BOX 4.10 Resources for medicines management**

- Interactive exercises on www.safeMedicate.com.
- British National Formulary (BNF) or BNF for Children online. If you are not already registered you can do so via www.medicinescomplete.com
- Revise the NMC (2008) Standards for Medicines Management www.nmc.org.uk/standards/additional-standards/standards-for-medicines-management/
- Undertake any supplementary records for medicines management.
- Complete competencies in your assessment of practice portfolio (AOP).

---

Please refer to Chapter 5, section "Medicines Management Practice Questions" where there are working examples of medication-related questions asked at interview.

## PSYCHOMETRIC AND APTITUDE TESTS

These techniques are commonplace in the business world; the purpose is to affirm whether or not the candidate's personality and aptitude are right for the vacancy. They are gaining in popularity in healthcare as screening tools. The biggest fears seem to be around the unknown element of the exam and the potential for "incorrect" answers on personality tests. *"What if I am not the person they are looking for?"*

There are five broad categories of test (Innes 2012b); however, it is the first three types that healthcare registrants are most likely to encounter:

1. Personality tests/questionnaires
2. Verbal reasoning
3. Numeracy/numerical reasoning
4. Spatial and diagrammatic reasoning
5. Clerical and data checking

The technique to answering these is to carefully read the question. In personality tests, such as the well-known Myers-Briggs Type Indicator (1962 cited in the Myers-Briggs Foundation 2014), there is no right or wrong answer and questions will be framed in such a way as to make it difficult to convince the interpreter that you are anyone other than your real self. To this end it is important to be honest.

In contrast, verbal reasoning is assessing a very clear skill set that is about information management. Responses will indicate how well a candidate understands, processes, analyses and interprets language. Spelling and grammar are also assessed components. There is much to be gained from practising questions; however, most institutions will keep papers a closely guarded secret.

Numerical competency is measured by means of simple mental calculations, patterns, sequencing, charts and graphs, none of which should require the use of a calculator (unless reasonable adjustment is indicated). Applicants who have a disability and believe that they may be disadvantaged by the use of psychometric tests are advised to consult the SHL (2005) best practice guidelines or seek advice from the Royal National Institute for the Blind (2012) and British Psychological Society Psychological Testing Centre (BPSPTC) guides for those with dyslexia (2006), hearing (2007) or visual impairment (2010).

Candidates again are encouraged to familiarise themselves with the formats of tests, in particular multi-choice question papers. Box 4.11 highlights a number of helpful resources.

---

**BOX 4.11 Resources for psychometric and aptitude tests**

- Innes (2012b, Chapter 14) – outline examples of the five main types (see above).
- Association of Graduate Careers Advisory Services Psychometric Assessment Test Group (PATG) (2015). Guidance on key psychometric assessment tools. This is available for HE careers services to use with graduates so it is worth asking at the university careers service.

- TARGETjobs – an introduction to psychometric tests with free practice tests and tips online at: http://targetjobs.co.uk/careers-advice/psychometric-tests/275677-psychometric-tests-what-they-are-and-why-graduates-need-to-know.
- Bryon (2012) Ultimate Psychometric Tests: Over 1000 Verbal Numerical Diagrammatic and IQ Practice Tests.
- Parkinson (2010) How to Master Psychometric Tests.
- Parkinson (2014) Psychometric Tests and University admissions tests. Heralded by UK Jobs Network as "The most comprehensive list of practice psychometric tests and questionnaires available on the web"; follow this link at www.markparkinson.co.uk/psychometric_links.htm.
- Free test papers can be found online at www.psychometric-success.com/index.htm.

## HOW TO GAIN YOUR OWN EXPERIENCE AS AN INTERVIEWER

Some undergraduate students will have gained valuable experience assisting on open days or taking part in the selection of prospective students for places on pre-registration nursing and midwifery programmes. If it is not too late, investigate opportunities that may exist in your HE institution so you can see, from the other side of the process, what a recruiter looks for and benefit from their expertise. Working in partnership with academic and clinical staff breaks down perceived boundaries and extends your network of contacts for the future.

You will need to work with the selection criteria and make judgements about an individual's suitability, based on what you know about the discipline, core values and what it takes to succeed to registration as a professional nurse or midwife. Whilst there will be standardised selection techniques (i.e. a set group interview activity or panel interviews), it is worth rotating between different selectors in order to gain a better understanding of best practice, any subtle variations in approach or focus and how several perspectives contribute to the decision-making process. Staff will support you in this role; you can ask them to write you a testimony for your AOP and you can also put this experience on your CV.

## APPLICATIONS, INTERVIEW CONDUCT AND THE LAW

All NHS employees, under the revised NHS Employment Check Standards (NHS Employers 2013), will be subject to six pre-employment checks. These are in relation to:

1.  Identity
2.  Right to work
3.  Professional registration and qualifications
4.  Employment history and references
5.  Criminal record and barring
6.  Work health assessments*

*The term "work health assessments" now replaces what were previously referred to as "occupational health checks". More information can be found on the NHS Employers website.

Every applicant has to be afforded the same opportunity and employers are bound by legislation when processing applications, interviewing prospective employees and offering posts. The key legislation that you need to know about is the following:

*   Equality Act 2010 for United Kingdom (except Northern Ireland)
*   Disability Discrimination Act 1995 (Northern Ireland Government) and the Disability Discrimination (NI) Order 2006 (DDO)
*   Border and Immigration Agency guidance for the appointment of non-EU Nationals
*   2 Tier Certificate of Sponsorship (formerly work permits)
*   The Rehabilitation of Offenders Act (Exceptions Order) 1975
*   The Disclosure and Barring Service (DBS) Check which applies to all candidates.

It is important to note that there is different legislation in Northern Ireland. Conduct associated with discrimination and the related legislation is summarised in Table 4.2.

This section will provide a brief overview; the highly complex and changing nature of some legislation means that some applicants may need expert advice which is beyond the remit of this book. At the end of this chapter there is a list of resources including the websites of professional bodies that can be contacted for further information.

| TABLE 4.2 Conduct associated with discrimination and related legislation ||
|---|---|
| **Area** | **Law** |
| Age discrimination | Equality Act 2010 |
| | The Employment Equality (Age) Regulations (Northern Ireland) 2006 |
| Sexual discrimination includes: | Equality Act 2010 |
| • Marital status (married, divorced, civil partnerships or same-sex marriage) | Employment Equality (Sex Discrimination) Regulations (Northern Ireland) 2005 |
| • Being pregnant or having a child | |
| • Gender | |
| • Sexual orientation | |
| • Being or becoming a transsexual | |
| Racial discrimination | Equality Act 2010 |
| • Ethnic background | Race Relations Order (Amendment) Regulations (Northern Ireland) 2003 |
| • Colour | |
| • Birthplace | |
| • Name | |
| • Nationality | |
| Religious discrimination on basis of: | Equality Act 2010 |
| • Appearance | Fair Employment and Treatment Order (Amendment ) Regulations (Northern Ireland) 2003 |
| • Belief/religion | |
| • Lack of belief/religion | |
| Disability discrimination | Equality Act 2010 |
| • A disabled person has the same rights as other workers. Employers should also make "reasonable adjustments" to help disabled employees and job applicants | Disability Discrimination Act 1995 Amended Regulations (Northern Ireland) 2004 |
| | Disability Discrimination (Northern Ireland) Order 2006 |
| Health | Equality Act 2010 |
| • Questions which are unrelated to the job role are unlawful | Disability Discrimination Act 1995 Amended Regulations (Northern Ireland) 2004 |
| • Cannot discriminate against those with medical conditions | Disability Discrimination (Northern Ireland) Order 2006 |
| • Reasonable adjustments again apply | Work Health Assessments (NHS Employers 2013) |
| | Data Protection Act 1998 |

| Area | Law |
|------|-----|
| **TABLE 4.2** *continued* | |
| Criminal convictions (essentially spent convictions) <br><br> • Disclosure and Barring Service (DBS) <br> www.gov.uk/disclosure-barring-service-check/overview | Rehabilitation of Offenders Act 2001 <br> Freedom of Information Act 2012 <br> Disclosure and Barring Service checks <br> The Public Interest Disclosure (Northern Ireland) Order 1998 |
| Trade Union <br><br> • Membership <br> • Non-membership | Equality Act 2010 |
| Type of employment <br><br> • Fixed term <br> www.gov.uk/fixed-term-contracts/employees-rights <br><br> • Part time <br> www.gov.uk/part-time-worker-rights | Equality Act 2010 <br> The Part-Time Workers (Prevention of Less Favourable Treatment) Regulations 2000 |

## THE EQUALITY ACT AND DDA (APPLIES TO NORTHERN IRELAND)

In general terms the Equality Act (Great Britain Parliament 2010) covers discrimination of "protected characteristics" and makes it unlawful for employers to discriminate on the grounds of "age, disability, gender reassignment, marriage and civil partnership, pregnancy and maternity, race, religion or belief, sex and sexual orientation". The Employment Statutory Code of Practice (Equality and Human Rights Commission (EHRC) 2010) is an authoritative guide for both employers and employees alike. In Northern Ireland employers and employees should refer to the Disability Discrimination Act (DDA) (1995) and Disability Discrimination (NI) Order 2006 (DDO).

In order to monitor compliance with the Equality Act (2010) NHS job applicants will be asked a number of mandatory questions. These appear under the section entitled "Monitoring Information" and relate to age, gender, ethnicity, sexual orientation, religion or belief and disability. This information is not made available to selectors during the shortlisting process. Selectors should be very clear about the law and adhere strictly to good practice to avoid legal action. Chapter 5 considers interview questions that are considered unlawful.

## DISABILITY OR HEALTH NEEDS

The guiding principle here is that role suitability overrides disability; therefore an employer should not treat an applicant with a disability any differently from other candidates. The person does not have to be registered disabled in order to be able to say they have a disability; a disability is classed as "a physical or mental impairment that has a 'substantial' and 'long-term' negative effect on your ability to do normal daily activities" (Office for Disability Issues (ODI) 2010). There is a wide spectrum of disability ranging from mental health conditions, dyslexia and dyspraxia, stammer, chronic fatigue syndrome, latex allergy to cancer, multiple sclerosis and HIV (all three of the latter at point of diagnosis). However, the term of reference does not include addiction to non-prescribed drugs or alcohol dependency.

There are a few specific circumstances when an interviewer can ask questions about health and disability during the initial stages of a recruitment process. This is explained in the Government Equalities Office guide (2011, p. 3–4). The six reasons are:

1. To establish whether the applicant can take part in an assessment to determine their suitability for the job
2. To determine whether any reasonable adjustments need to be made to enable a disabled person to participate in an assessment during the recruitment process
3. To find out whether a job applicant would be able to undertake a function that is intrinsic to the job
4. To support "positive action" in employment for disabled people
5. To monitor diversity among job applicants
6. If there is an occupational requirement for disabled applicants

For example in relation to reason number 3, this would apply in a role where moving and handling is an intrinsic element. The employer therefore can ask if an applicant has any health or disability that prevents them from fulfilling the job. However, at the same time an employer cannot ask about previous sickness absence.

That said, if a candidate declares a disability on an application and this requires "reasonable adjustments" then the employer must accommodate the request. To get the adjustment, they may reasonably be asked to provide evidence of the condition and its effect from a doctor or registered professional such as an educational psychologist. Examples would include a person with dyslexia needing extra time to complete exams or someone who requires regular breaks during a long interview schedule to effectively manage their diabetes. Conversely, if a candidate chooses not to declare a disability or health need on the application form, they cannot expect the benefit from modifications in the assessment process. In addition an applicant who withholds information about a disability could arguably be disadvantaged because they do not appear to meet requirements under the category of "positive action" (see section "Positive Action").

At the point of a job offer, or when an applicant is placed in a pool of successful applicants to be offered jobs as vacancies arise, a conditional offer will be made. This means that the offer is subject to the individual meeting the employer's health or other requirements. Thereafter the Equality Act (2010) does not restrict the employer asking questions regarding health or disability. From the employer's perspective it is important to know whether a successful applicant is eligible for job-related benefits or requires reasonable adjustments to enable them to do the job. A final job award decision should not discriminate against disabled people (Government Equalities Office 2011).

## POSITIVE ACTION

An employer may encourage applicants from under-represented groups such as black and ethnic minority (BME) groups through "positive actions" (Point 16.29 EHRC 2010); this is not the same as positive discrimination, which is unlawful. An example would be restricting recruitment to a specific BME group (i.e. Bangladeshi) for a post where they may require language proficiency and cultural awareness. The same might apply to posts targeting older people or those with a disability where seniority or disability is viewed as additional qualifications.

Furthermore, Point 12.32 states that an employer would not be acting unlawfully if they have a policy for interviewing all disabled applicants providing that they meet the minimum requirements for the job that are essential but not desirable components. An example of this is on NHS Jobs applications where there are two tick boxes:

- If you have a disability, do you require any reasonable adjustments to be made during the recruitment process, including interview? If so please give details (box provided).
- If you have a disability, do you wish to be considered under the Guaranteed Interview Scheme if you meet the minimum criteria as specified in the Person Specification?

The RCN Peer Support Service (part of the Member Support Services 0345 408 4391) provides emotional support to nurses who have a disability and offers help to anyone who has experienced discrimination and those wishing to return to work after injury or illness.

## EXCEPTIONS

There are a few exceptions to the rules about discrimination. One is if it is a genuine occupational requirement (GOR) (Innes 2012b; HM Government 2013a); a case being work within a religious order where religious affiliation is essential. In the same way a women's refuge that lawfully provides services to vulnerable women would require all its staff to be female. The other exception relates to the armed services who are exempt from some elements of employment legislation.

## WORK HEALTH ASSESSMENTS (FORMERLY OCCUPATIONAL HEALTH CHECKS)

All applicants will be subject to a pre-employment work health assessment. Every NHS organisation across England must comply with the new Work Health Assessment (WHA) checks (NHS Employers 2013) which take into account the Equality Act (2010), the Data Protection Act (Great Britain Parliament 1998) and good occupational health practice. The WHA document provides a succinct overview of the standards relating to health assessment and disability (i.e. what can and what cannot be asked on applications and at interview), disclosure, the process of occupational health checks and what constitutes reasonable adjustment (e.g. altering working hours, special equipment). Refusal of employment can only be made after the following:

- Expert occupational medical advice has been sought
- The applicant has had the opportunity to discuss issues raised with an occupational health provider
- The employing manager has given full consideration to all of the facts (NHS Employers 2013, p. 8)

Again honesty is paramount. If certain aspects of the role would adversely affect health (for example, undertaking night duty presents risks to an individual who has epilepsy) this is as much about preventing risk to the individual employee. If you are unsure about whether or not you should disclose information, you need to ask yourself whether or not the health condition or disability might affect your work and as a result you might require special adjustments to either your anticipated work or place of work.

## BORDER AND IMMIGRATION AGENCY GUIDANCE FOR THE APPOINTMENT OF NON-EU NATIONALS

Non-EU nationals need to familiarise themselves with the latest Border and Immigration Agency guidance. Employers are legally bound to work within this. Due to the changing nature of legislation, you must refer to the most up-to-date information. Applying for work, sponsorship and residency take time and can be costly so it is important to start the process early, use professional advice and make contingency plans.

For registrants there are a number of key sources of information:

- Home Office UK Border Agency (UKBA) website:
  - www.ukba.homeoffice.gov.uk/visas-immigration/
- Nursing and Midwifery Council (NMC)
  - www.nmc-uk.org/Registration/Joining-the-register/
  - Choose from one of three options: trained in UK; trained in Europe; trained outside Europe
  - Non-EU nationals should refer to the NMC (2012b) document called "Registering as a nurse or midwife in the United Kingdom (for applicants from countries outside of the European Economic Area)"
- NHS Careers website for information about the Points-Based System (PBS) for assessing immigration applications for the UK www.nhscareers.nhs.uk
- The RCN Immigration Advice Service (IAS) immigration.advice@rcn. org.uk Telephone: 0345 408 4391 (option 1). Provides free confidential advice and assistance with:
  - Points-Based System (PBS)
    - Tier 2 (skilled workers)
    - Tier 4 (students)
    - Tier 5 (temporary workers i.e. HCAs/youth mobility scheme applicants)
  - Change or extension of current visa
  - Marriage and Civil Partnership Applications
  - Indefinite Leave to Remain (ILR) (Settlement) Applications
  - British Citizenship through Naturalisation and Registration
  - European Economic Area (EEA) national queries

It is helpful to know that the RCN advice is available to non-members (nursing staff from overseas, nursing students and HCAs in the UK) who are currently not eligible for membership.

- Non-EU migrant workers who are also UNISON members can get advice on immigration issues related to employment and the right to work in the UK on 0800 0 857 857 or visit www.unison.org.uk/knowledge/pay/migrant-workers/overview/#7.
- Royal College of Midwives: The RCM does not have any specific document or adviser in relation to advice for non-EU midwives who wish to register in the UK. Midwives should visit the NMC website (see above) as all the information they require is available there.

In 2008 a new Points-Based System (PBS) was introduced for assessing immigration applications for the UK (NHS Jobs 2014). There are five tiers spanning temporary to highly skilled workers. The number of points required for each tier varies; applicants gain points according to their qualifications, experience, age, previous earnings and language proficiency. On this system, university students from outside the UK or EEA will be tier 4; they will require a visa which allows them to undertake part-time work during term time and full-time work during holiday periods. Tier 2 (skilled workers) includes registered nurses and midwives. This system allows NHS organisations the ability to employ non-EEA nationals when they cannot fill vacancies with a British or EEA worker. There will be some specialisms on the skills shortage list (i.e. neonatal intensive care) deemed as priority areas for overseas recruitment; however, the employing body must satisfy the Resident Labour Market test to show that there are no suitable EU/EEA candidates. The employer has to apply to the UKBA for a Certificate of Sponsorship for each applicant they sponsor. The UKBA will not grant Indefinite Leave to Remain or British Citizenship to anyone with unspent criminal convictions.

## DISCLOSURE AND BARRING SERVICE (DBS) CHECK (FORMERLY KNOWN AS CRB)

Nursing and midwifery posts are subject to the Rehabilitation of Offenders Act (Exceptions Order) 1975 and as such it will be necessary for a submission for disclosure to be made to the Disclosure and Barring Service (formerly known as CRB) to check for any previous criminal convictions. This is an enhanced criminal record check to include "any information which may be held against the barred list for working with children and/or adults" (NHS Jobs 2014).

This means that nurses and midwives must disclose both spent and unspent criminal convictions. If an applicant fails either intentionally or recklessly to disclose information relating to any convictions this could lead to the withdrawal of a job offer, dismissal, disciplinary action and referral to the NMC. On the NHS Jobs application form there is a section marked "Criminal Convictions" which asks applicants two questions; if you answer yes you must include details. You will also be asked if you have any penalty points on your driving licence; if so how many, the Endorsement Offence Codes and date of issue. However, you do not need to disclose parking offences.

In summary, employment law is complex. Further advice on interpreting the law should be obtained from:

- ACAS (Advisory, Conciliation and Arbitration Service) Helpline 08457 47 47 47 for free support and advice or to check workplace policies and practices. This helpline provides impartial advice for employers and employees on a range of employment relations, employment rights, and HR and management issues.
- NHS Employers website: www.nhsemployers.org/RECRUITMENT ANDRETENTION/EMPLOYMENT-CHECKS/Pages/Employment-checks.aspx.
- Northern Ireland Government website: www.nidirect.gov.uk/definition-of-disability.
- Equality Commission for Northern Ireland website: www.equalityni.org.
- HM Government Working, Jobs and Pensions on www.gov.uk/browse/working.
- A local job centre.

# 5

# Preparing for Interview

## KEY WORDS

Logistics; personal safety; documentation; mental preparation; background research; mock questions; STAR/ CAR frameworks; dress codes; nerves; first impressions; what to avoid; asking questions; managing success/rejection; dilemmas

You have been invited for an interview, which is great news! The next hurdle puts you firmly in the spotlight in every sense and the amount of preparation needed should not be underestimated. This section will take time to remind you of what might seem like the basics but will really make a positive difference to your performance on the day. Whilst respecting that many students have had other careers before becoming nurses and midwives and thereby have prior interview experience, there will be some distinct differences in nursing and midwifery interviews. For example, you may have had placements in the area that you are applying to, you may know members of the interview panel and this time you will probably know fellow students who are applying for the same NQN/NQM posts. This is no time for complacency.

## DATE AND TIME

There are few reasons why you would not accept the date and time offered. Exceptions would include:

- A clash with another interview which you have already accepted (unless of course you then cancel it)
- Funerals, weddings or jury service
- Urgent dental or hospital appointments that cannot be rescheduled

As soon as you receive the invitation you should formally acknowledge this in writing or with a phone call. If you are unable to attend you should explain why. In the event that there is no alternative date, you could ask whether you could be interviewed by phone or webcam instead.

## CONTACT DETAILS

The invitation should provide you with a key contact for correspondence. This may not be one of the people who will be interviewing, so you need to ascertain who you will meet on the day and their respective job titles. This forms part of your preparatory homework.

## LOCATION AND PERSONAL SAFETY

There are good reasons for taking time to find out more about the location, particularly if you are going somewhere unfamiliar. Traffic congestion or problems with public transport will not be accepted as an excuse for lateness. The only reasonable exception would be flight or train cancellation or delay due to unforeseen circumstances (e.g. extreme weather conditions, flooding or a major accident or incident). If this happens it is important to contact the recruiter as soon as you can to explain this and discuss a solution if you cannot attend in person. Plan to arrive at the venue at least 30–45 minutes before you are required. An early interview may necessitate travelling there the day before and an overnight stay close to the venue so you can be confident that you will be there on time.

Your primary contact or the HR department can provide information on local parking facilities. Alternatively look on their website. It is important to factor in sufficient time for parking; there may be limited parking at peak times when there are busy outpatient clinics or it is visiting time. Interviews may run over so you should not use on-street parking which is time-restricted, that is, 1 hour maximum parking. A better option, and one that can significantly reduce your stress levels, is to ask someone else to drive you to the interview, to drop you off and to collect you so you do not have to worry about parking especially if it will be dark when the interview finishes. Personal safety is paramount; always tell someone where you are going and call them when the interview has finished. Candidates should never agree to being interviewed in premises other than the organisation's or a public place; nor should they accept an interviewer's offer of a lift (Innes 2012b).

## SPECIAL REQUIREMENTS

Applicants who require reasonable adjustments (as discussed in Chapters 3 and 4) again must make the recruiter aware in advance. Furthermore, if the selection process includes a catered break and you have a special dietary requirement then you must advise them accordingly.

## DOCUMENTATION

In addition to your assessment of practice portfolio (AOP), start to collate information in a dedicated folder. This should include:

- Interview invitation
- Directions/maps and parking instructions

- Your application form
- Job description and person specification
- All documents associated with the job vacancy and employer (see Table 5.1)
- Professional certificates
- NMC PIN (plastic card)
- Passport
- Valid driving licence
- Disclosure and Barring Service (DBS) certificate (formerly known as CRB)
- Work permit/visas
- A set of 6–8 questions to ask the recruiters

Invest time in collating and tagging any documents you intend to refer to in the interview. Presentation matters and should be to a high standard; failure to do so will convey a lack of attention to detail. The employer may ask to see and take copies of key documents.

## MENTAL PREPARATION

Having passed the initial selection process and secured an interview you then move into the next highly competitive phase of the process. Ideally you will have begun your preparations in anticipation of being offered an interview; however, take a moment to congratulate yourself and reflect. If you could capture this feeling what would it be? Pride? A sense of achievement and increased self-belief? To be shortlisted you need to have met the person specification and thereby selectors believe that you may be the right person for the job. The interview environment will put to the test your ability to sell yourself and give you an opportunity to secure a favourable outcome. Nerves, misplaced modesty and poor preparation can undermine how you project yourself; conversely candidates who stretch the truth and are overconfident will be identified and potentially challenged by a skilful interviewer.

A good night's sleep before an interview is important. Unless under medical supervision, do not self-medicate with any drugs that may impair your performance. Consider rearranging your off-duty and other commitments to ensure that you have adequate time to physically and mentally prepare yourself on the day of the interview.

## BACKGROUND RESEARCH

Preparation is essential and will pay dividends. Table 5.1 provides a list of the key areas to focus your background research on. Given the ease with which you can access electronic information, an employer will expect an applicant to have a sound understanding of the organisation they wish to work for, including the type of services they provide, their mission statement and values, key policy directives as well as the job itself. If there are attachments within the advert or webpages that you are signposted to, it is essential that you download all the relevant documents. An appreciation of other more practical issues such as location and parking will help you identify potential problems and plan strategies to ensure you arrive with plenty of time to spare. Work through the list and keep notes/printouts for reference.

| TABLE 5.1 My interview to-do list | |
| --- | --- |
| **Background** | **Tick** |
| • Employer. <br> • Look at website (location, services, facilities, future plans for the organisation, employee benefits and HR). <br> • Obtain a contact name in the department/area of interest. <br> • Organise an informal visit prior to interview. <br> • Ask employees. <br> • Read annual reports (Trust; CQC) and institution's research. <br> • Print off trust values – you will need these for your personal statement. <br> • Think about personal safety if you will be working shifts, commuting or visiting clients on your own in the community. | |
| **The role** | |
| • Print off the job description, person specification and any attachments within these documents or the main advert itself (i.e. summary of terms and conditions and information regarding previous criminal convictions). The amount of information will vary. <br> • Print off your application. <br> • Use a highlighter to make key words stand out. <br> • Make notes in relation to the core job requirements. <br> • Be clear how your skills and experience match requirements. <br> • Identify how you meet the trust's values. <br> • Choose real examples from practice to illustrate abilities. | |

**TABLE 5.1** *continued*

- Update your knowledge and skills on specialist aspects of the role.
- Identify current issues and read around the topic areas.
- Refer to key policy documents that are relevant to the role and area of practice, that is, safeguarding, mental capacity, moving and handling and infection control.

**Rehearse**

- Organise pre-interview practice with either
  - A critical friend
  - Your university careers adviser
  - Your tutor group
- Draw up a list of possible questions (refer to the lists in section "Practice Questions").
- Prepare for other selection methods (i.e. psychometric tests and role play).
- Reflect on your strengths and weaknesses and continue practicing.
- Draw up six to eight questions you want to ask the interviewer (refer to Table 5.2, p. 128). Think carefully about the order and if you are not sure about the appropriateness of a question, ask for advice beforehand.

## MOCK QUESTIONS

The questions in Activity 5.1 are based on real questions asked at interviews. Rehearsing your answers will force you to think about both the structure and content of your answers, what you need to emphasise and suitable illustrations. You can set up a mock interview with your tutor and peers, a careers adviser or critical friend; they will give feedback not just on detail but importantly on your overall performance. One successful student said, "I had a mock interview at the careers service and it was so helpful and prepared me for the interview. It also got me into the right mind set as I had not had one for 3 years. The guidance and support ensured that I could carry out further preparation such as more reading. I believe the mock interview prepared me enough to get the job."

It is worth making notes as prompts and identifying any topics which you need to look into further. Use post-its around the house to help you remember key points and transpose these onto crib cards that can discretely be referred to in a waiting area. Experience shows that, in the heat of the moment, candidates often forget the most obvious, for example, to explicitly talk about their *accountability* (NMC 2015a). This is one key word that all interviewers will be expecting to hear, so perhaps a discrete "A" penned onto your hand will be a timely reminder to you when you are under pressure.

Start practicing with a few warm-up questions (Activity 5.1). Introductory questions can be asked for a number of the following reasons:

- To put you at ease
- To help you connect with the panel
- To provide an early chance to impress panel members
- To catch the unprepared interviewee off guard either because they cannot think of an answer to a routine question, and dry up, or conversely start talking and stray from the point

---

**ACTIVITY 5.1**

**Role play common warm-up questions**

You have applied for a job where you had a clinical placement 2 months ago. You have been encouraged by the staff to apply ("they want me back as a newly qualified"). These are the warm-up questions asked by the panel:

**Question A**  "How was your journey here today?"
**Question B**  "Tell us about yourself."
**Question C**  "What have you really enjoyed in your nursing/midwifery course?"

1. Write down how you would initially answer each one.
2. Before you read an answer out, revisit the question and ask yourself, "What is the interviewer looking for in my response?"
3. Amend your answer accordingly.
4. Now stand in front of a mirror and rehearse your answer until you feel you can give a confident and natural response.
5. Then ask a friend to ask you these questions.

Ask them to give you constructive feedback on the way in which you answered the questions. This is about delivery as well as content.

Now compare your answers for questions A–C with the following model answers.

**Question A**  "How was your journey here today?"
**Reply**       "Fine. Thank you. I did not encounter any problems because I gave myself ample time and the directions you provided were very helpful."

**Displays**     Good time management, reference to pre-interview instructions and courtesy.

**Question B**   "Tell me about yourself."

**Reply**        "I am a final year student on the Nursing degree programme. I have always wanted a career as a children's nurse. After college I took a gap year, initially to travel but I was very fortunate to find a volunteering opportunity and spent 6 months working in a special school in Inner London with children who have physical and developmental disabilities. In my spare time I play hockey for the University Ladies team and work for NHS Professionals."

**Displays**     Motivation, experience, diverse interests, values and personality.

**Question C**   "What have you really enjoyed about your midwifery course?"

**Reply**        "Initially I felt very conscious that I had limited work experience before I started the programme. However as soon as we started to learn about maternal health and I had my first placement I realised I had made completely the right career choice. Each placement has been very different. My confidence has grown parallel with the acquisition of new skills and knowledge. I have relished every opportunity to engage with practitioners, women and their partners and to be involved in delivering babies and postnatal care. I feel my role gives me a privileged position at a critical time in people's lives and I have enjoyed being part of some amazing experiences like the delivery of twins and my first home birth. I've always felt part of the team and this has supported me when I have felt under pressure and in need of advice. I am a high achiever and I have really pushed myself hard to achieve good grades both in practice and academic work."

**Displays**     Passion for the discipline and a career in midwifery, motivation, valuing partnership and team working and seeing learning as integral to development.

Moving beyond the introduction, there are many broad-based questions that can be asked and of course it is impossible to rehearse for every eventuality. An interviewer may use questions that focus on what you have done, rather than how you might respond to a scenario. The purpose of this is to gain concrete and verifiable evidence about your readiness for a role. These types of questions are known as behavioural interview questions. These are the questions that ask you to explain a situation in which you demonstrated a certain skill. For example, "Tell me about an occasion when your action made a positive impact on the care of an individual." The key is to identify suitable past experiences to use as examples.

## HOW TO CONSTRUCT A GOOD ANSWER

Applying the well-known STAR or CAR frameworks will help you build a comprehensive answer to any situational question you may face. **STAR** stands for **S**ituation; **T**ask, **A**ction and **R**esult and is widely used in competency-based interviewing. **CAR** is about **C**ontext, **A**ction and **R**esult and is easier to remember in a pressurised situation. Refer to Box 5.1.

### BOX 5.1 The CAR framework

**Context/Challenge:**
- Describe the situation.
- Describe the task.
- When and where was this?
- Who was with **YOU**?

**Action:**
- What action did **YOU** take?
- Do not focus on the contributions of others and remember that the interviewer wants to hear about **YOUR** individual contribution.

**Results:**
- What positive results did **YOU** achieve?
- What conclusions did **YOU** reach?
- What did **YOU** learn from the experience?

**C** can also stand for **C**hallenge (Vanderbilt University 2014) or **C**ircumstances; none are wrong so choose whichever one you prefer. All will help you craft a succinct and accurate description of an issue or opportunity where you showed initiative. Again this last element is about *you* and should always focus on the positive; selecting appropriate examples is therefore crucial. If you do not have work experience to match then you should not fake it.

The following example shows you how to use CAR to answer this question:
"Can you give an example of when you have demonstrated strong team-working skills?"

Answer:

**Context/Challenge:** This example is taken from my last placement which was with a community nursing *team*, I had responsibility for a caseload of patients. This usually meant six to eight visits a day, the majority of which I conducted on my own. On one occasion I had to ask for urgent assistance. This was when an elderly lady who had COPD had deteriorated suddenly and I needed my mentor to assess her.

**Action:** *I called* the office and explained the situation; my mentor was able to attend and after liaison with the GP, a decision was taken to admit this lady. *I took responsibility* for collating the lady's records and calling ahead to the respiratory ward to give them essential information. Throughout the process we supported the lady and her husband who was also frail. *I phoned* her daughter to tell her about her admission. The couple received daily input from a care agency so *I also contacted* social services to alert them to her admission and ensure that her husband's needs were noted.

**Results:** This *teamwork* meant the lady received prompt referral and admission. Because her husband was well-supported, this reduced some of the patient's anxiety. *My call* to the ward meant the staff were able to prepare for her admission. *It really emphasised to me* how important teamwork and good communication between different services is for patients like this lady. Despite the fact that she is in and out of hospital on a regular basis, every episode creates a major upset for this couple – you could see how traumatic and unsettling this was. *I was able to demonstrate my ability* to work as part of the wider team and thereby ensure a safe handover of care. Here is the report that my mentor wrote that relates to this skill." (Give example from portfolio to support.)

If you have evidence by way of testimonials and mentor reports, tagging these in your portfolio will enable you to quickly locate them to show the interviewer. Activity 5.2 gives you the opportunity to practice using the CAR technique yourself.

---

**ACTIVITY 5.2**

**Putting the CAR framework into practice**

Using the CAR framework, map out and rehearse your answer for the following questions:

1. Describe a time when you were able to improve the care of a client.
2. Can you tell me about a situation at work when you showed you could handle pressure and stress?
3. Give an example of when you have received negative feedback; how did you respond?
4. Can you give me an example of when you have successfully supported a junior student?

---

Fundamentally the real question behind every question is "Why should we employ you?". Listening to the question is essential as there is always the risk you have misheard and then proceed to give a pre-rehearsed answer to a question you think you have been asked.

## INTERVIEW FORMAT

If the interview invitation does not stipulate the format, it would be reasonable to seek clarification so you can rehearse accordingly. Video- and telephone-based interviews were discussed in Chapter 4, section "Telephone or Video Interviews".

If you are subject to a panel interview, it is important to direct your response to the person asking the question, whilst also making eye contact with other panel members. This is a technique that often requires practice, because people tend to have a dominant side (left or right) which means they turn and talk towards that side to the detriment of anyone standing or sitting on the other side. Arguably this is influenced by the personalities involved, any prior dealings with individuals and whether one person dominates the process. Nonetheless, when you are in next in a group situation such as during a handover, in a meeting or giving a presentation to peers, reflect on where you are positioned, whether or not you are drawn in a particular direction and if so are you inadvertently ignoring colleagues within the room? Panel members will be introduced to you at the start of the interview, by name and by title, so you know where they fit into the organisational structure. If name badges are visible or you can remember the names of those without a visible badge, then use this to personalise the reply.

Box 5.2 contains an account written by a student after his first interview.

---

**BOX 5.2 The applicant's perspective**

**Oscar:** This was a straightforward face-to-face interview for an NQN post on an older persons mental health ward. There were three people on the panel; the charge nurse, the unit manager and a lady from HR. It was far more formal than any previous interview I've had. I was asked:

- How and why would you grant Section 17 leave?
- What would you do if a patient's relative was being disruptive on the ward? Towards a patient? Towards staff?
- Can you give me an example of when you demonstrated your management and leadership skills?
- How would you prioritise your workload when you come on a shift?

I was really glad I'd taken my AOP with me and tagged important sections. They were keen to examine it and asked me what I'd gained in particular from my community and elective placement with the Homeless Link project. They spent time looking at my Personal Development Plan and questioning me about my ambitions. Thankfully I'd thought about where I want to be in 3 years' time."

---

## PRACTICE QUESTIONS

The following bank of sample questions is divided into generic and field-specific. The generic ones are suitable for both nursing and midwifery students to use to rehearse answers. The field ones have been provided by specialists within the relevant disciplines and also by former students. Service users have also provided a set of questions, again broken down into generic and discipline. Section "Medicines Management Practice Questions" contains generic and field-specific medicines management questions.

### GENERIC QUESTIONS FOR NURSING AND MIDWIFERY

1. Why do you want to work for this trust/organisation?
2. What attracted you to this particular area/specialism?
3. Tell me about yourself.
4. What have you gained from your degree programme?

5. What did you find most challenging on your course?
6. What skills would you bring to this department?
7. What would your clients say about you?
8. What are the best and worst things about your specialist area?
9. What comes first, clients or paperwork?
10. What are your key strengths and weaknesses?
11. When you are qualified, how will you keep yourself up to date?
12. Can you explain what is meant by the term "evidence-based practice" and give an example of how you use evidence to underpin your clinical practice?
13. What is your understanding of "clinical governance"?
14. How do the values of the NHS Constitution/this trust's values guide your practice?
15. Can you give a concise overview of what the 6Cs mean to you?
16. What do you consider to be the key issues affecting the profession today? Tell me about one of these issues (e.g. clinical governance, evidence-based practice, implications of the Francis Report, the Kirkup Report, the Dalton Review, the NHS Five Year Forward View, etc.).
17. Aside from financial issues, what do you think are the main issues that this trust is currently focused on?
18. Please describe your understanding of the term "clinical supervision" in relation to your practice and how you see this linking with the clinical governance agenda.
19. How do you switch off after a hard day at work?
20. Are there any reasons why you would not be able to move or handle patients with the appropriate training, equipment or resources?
21. What three things do you wish to achieve in your first year of employment?
22. What can the trust do to support you in your new role?
23. What do you know about our induction/preceptorship programme?
24. What are your long-term goals?
25. Give an example of when you have demonstrated strong team-working skills.
26. Give an example of when you have received negative feedback; how did you respond?
27. Describe a time when you were able to improve the care of a client.
28. If you witnessed a senior member of staff raising their voice to a client, what would you do?
29. You are asked by the ward manager to undertake a task that you have not previously undertaken. What is your response?
30. What role does a person with a long-term condition have in guiding their own care?

31. What do you understand by the term "expert patient" or "expert carer"?

## ADULT NURSING FIELD QUESTIONS

1.  How would you describe the role of a Band 5 nurse in the department?
2.  How would you care for someone after a head injury?
3.  You have made a drugs error; what would you do?
4.  What would you do if a patient's BP was 80/40?
5.  You have just found a patient who has fallen on the floor; what do you do?
6.  What would you do if one of your patients went missing?

## COMMUNITY AND PRIMARY CARE SETTING QUESTIONS

1.  What do you think are the main challenges for a nurse working in a community setting?
2.  How do you see the future for community nursing?
3.  Who are the key stakeholders you will come across working in the community?
4.  How would you challenge poor practice?
5.  You are concerned about the practice of another health professional (nursing or medical). How would you manage this?
6.  You are visiting an elderly patient at home who lives with their son/daughter and you become suspicious that they are withholding money/food/care from them. What would you do?
7.  You are visiting a patient who is terminally ill and wishes to die at home. They have young children at home who are clearly distressed by the situation. What would you do?
8.  You have identified your development needs in your new role at interview but these are regularly and consistently not being met. What would you do?

## CHILD NURSING FIELD QUESTIONS

1.  What are some of the key issues in family-centred care?
2.  You notice that a child in your care has bruises on her arm. What would your course of action be?
3.  You have an asthmatic child coming in and you are going to prepare the bedside. What would your course of action be?

4. How would you deal with a hysterical child in a ward?
5. A parent of a child is upset with the treatment the child is receiving. What would you do to rectify this situation?
6. How would you define confidentiality?
7. Discuss the advantages/disadvantages of respite care for children.

## LEARNING DISABILITIES NURSING FIELD

1. When working with a person with a learning disability how would a person-centred approach enhance inter-professional engagement?
2. How would you develop a care plan for a person with a learning disability?
3. How do you see learning disability nursing developing in the future?
4. How would you work with someone who has a learning disability and whose behaviour is escalating?
5. How would you deal with a situation where a family was hindering their son or daughter with a learning disability in terms of their development and independence?
6. What is your role in determining if a person with a learning disability is able to give consent?

## MENTAL HEALTH NURSING FIELD QUESTIONS

1. What do you believe would be the most challenging aspect of working in the mental health field?
2. Does a regular routine have any benefits for adults with mental health problems?
3. What do you know about the Mental Capacity Act?
4. You are told that a patient is "unresponsive and pasty". What do you do?
5. Should adults with mental health problems and a history of challenging behaviour be cared for in the community?
6. What changes in behaviour might be associated with a resident becoming depressed?
7. Discuss a piece of research you have undertaken or read about recently.

## MIDWIFERY QUESTIONS

1. What do you see as the main issues facing midwives at present?
2. Can you tell the panel about a piece of midwifery research that you have recently read? How has it influenced your work?

3. How would you cope if you were caring for a woman who experienced a still birth?
4. What qualities does a midwife need?
5. What is your understanding of the role of the midwife within child protection?
6. How would you offer education/support to a 15-year-old who is not engaging with midwifery services?
7. Can you outline the public health responsibilities of a midwife, for example, in relation to smoking, alcohol or breastfeeding?
8. Who do you feel should be present at a woman's birth? And should midwives influence this?

## GENERIC QUESTIONS ASKED BY SERVICE USERS

1. How would you ensure your own prejudices and stigmas do not interfere with offering compassionate treatment?
2. Why is service user participation important and how would you champion this within your role?
3. Drawing on your placement experience, why is it important to involve service users?
4. How would you preserve your own emotional well-being whilst working in a stressful environment?
5. What do service user/patient-led outcomes mean to you?
6. Can you tell me about an occasion when you acted as an advocate for a vulnerable client?
7. How do you respond to the service user who invites you to be their Facebook friend?
8. I have let you into my home and my life; how will you show me that I can trust you?
9. Can you tell me why you want to be a registered nurse/midwife?
10. Can you tell us how your placement experience has developed your understanding of yourself, as a nurse/midwife?

## ADULT FIELD QUESTION FROM A SERVICE USER

When you have a busy caseload, how can you make an individual patient feel like they are important and not just part of a conveyer belt?

## CHILD FIELD QUESTION FROM A SERVICE USER

What are the rights of children and young people and how would you promote these within your role?

## LEARNING DISABILITIES FIELD QUESTION FROM A SERVICE USER

What interests you about working with young people with learning difficulties?

## MENTAL HEALTH FIELD QUESTIONS FROM A SERVICE USER

1.  What interests you about working with young people with mental health difficulties?
2.  What are the rights of children and young people and how would you promote these within your role?
3.  Sometimes mental health nurses are not welcome in people's homes. How would you manage this scenario?

## MIDWIFERY QUESTIONS FROM A SERVICE USER

1.  Midwifery can be very demanding. How do you cope under pressure?
2.  Why do you think it is important for midwives to be aware of diversity issues?

## MEDICINES MANAGEMENT PRACTICE QUESTIONS

Again these questions, generic and field-specific, are for you to use to rehearse.

1.  What drugs can be administered at the discretion of a nurse or midwife?
2.  What is a PGD and who can administer it?
3.  What are the six rights of medicines administration that a nurse/ midwife has to think about in the moment of giving a drug?
4.  What would you do if a patient refused their medication?
5.  Is covert administration of drugs acceptable?
6.  What would you do if you made a drug error?
7.  If a client was prescribed 7.5mg of a drug, how many 3.75mg tablets would you give?
8.  Convert 0.5mg to mcg.
9.  A patient has been prescribed 1 litre of normal saline to be run over 8 hours. How many millilitres an hour should the infusion be administered?

10. **Adult field:** What dose of enoxaparin should be prescribed for a 75 kg female patient needing treatment for a pulmonary embolism (PE) at 1.5mg/kg?
11. **Child field:** A child weighing 12 kg needs a treatment dose of iron for anaemia at 6mg/kg/day. What volume of Sytron liquid should the child be prescribed? Note that Sytron liquid contains 27.5 mg iron in 5 mls.
12. **Mental health field:** A client is prescribed an anti-psychotic depot. They refuse. As their primary nurse what would you do?
13. **Learning disabilities field:** How would you support someone with a learning disability to take their medication at the prescribed time?
14. **Midwifery:** With the direct supervision of a midwife the student should be involved in administering prescribed medicines (with the exception of controlled drugs) via which of the following routes?
    a) Oral
    b) Inhaled
    c) Central venous cannula
    d) Flushing lines with transducers
    e) Intramuscular

## HOW TO PRESENT YOURSELF ON THE DAY

This section considers dress codes, how to allay nerves, what to do if you are late and questions you may wish to ask the interviewing panel.

### DRESS CODES FOR INTERVIEW

Here is a subject which is bound to cause a degree of angst, indecision and divided opinion. Most employers expect to see candidates smartly presented, with minimal fashion piercings or tattoos visible. Likewise make-up, perfume and aftershave in moderation and definitely no gum! Choosing in advance and rehearsing in your interview attire will help to reduce stress on the actual day of your interview. Whilst the need to create a professional impression is vital, so is comfort. Ill-fitting shoes may hinder your entry and indeed exit from the room; too short a skirt, a plunging neckline or lack of tie may leave you feeling awkward and exposed in front of a panel of recruiters. On a very practical note, if you have a distance to walk, put your smart interview shoes in a bag and wear something more comfortable like trainers for the commute. If you envisage being taken on a tour of the unit or hospital as part of the inter-view process then think carefully about the suitability of your footwear.

Conservative dress (what your grandmother may approve of) is usually the safer bet. This should not incur excessive cost; some of the best-dressed applicants have found sale and charity shop bargains or borrowed a suit. Again it is wise to seek a second opinion regarding your choice. Some elements of dress may be dictated by cultural or religious norms which recruiters will take into account. However, feedback from recruiters suggests that wearing flip-flops, an outfit more suited for night clubbing, and taking a dependant (child) to interview definitely left a lasting and negative impression!

## THE LATE ARRIVAL

"I'm late! I'm late! For a very important date! No time to say hello, goodbye! I'm late! I'm late! I'm late!" sang the White Rabbit, in the film adaptation of Alice's Adventures in Wonderland (Lewis Carroll 1865).

In summary you have more than likely missed the boat! You could be 10 minutes late and still interview well, but less than half of recruiters questioned would offer you a job (Innes 2012b). One candidate with glowing references was late because he went to the wrong department by mistake; interviewers doubted his ability to follow instructions under pressure.

## DEALING WITH YOUR NERVES

So you are on time, in fact at least 30 minutes early, and you have located the reception area. You want to create a positive impression from the moment you enter the door, so here are a few tips you can practice.

- Take a deep breath, shoulders back, head up.
- Think how you will introduce yourself.
- Think about the value of small talk. Do not complain about the parking or the unhelpful staff; instead stick to a safe topic such as the weather.
- The recruiter may ask the receptionist for their impression of you.
- Switch off your mobile phone; do not sit in the reception area talking or texting.

Whilst you are waiting outside the interview room there are some key considerations:

- Will you sit or stand? An upright chair may improve your posture and composure, whereas a comfy chair encourages slouching and potentially projects a casual impression.

- Read! A clinical journal will create a better impression than a glossy magazine.
- A set of prompt cards with key words, that is, *accountability* and *EBP* with outline examples.
- Keep taking deep breaths and focus on being calm.
- Think about a positive clinical experience, that is, one where you were praised for the care you gave and one which left you feeling valued and self-confident.
- Refer back to the good feeling you had when you were offered the interview.
- Interviews may be delayed or take longer than anticipated. Drinking too much caffeine-based refreshment may play havoc on an already nervous bladder.

## ENTERING THE INTERVIEW ROOM

Impressions and etiquette continue to count as you move into the interview itself. After all and despite your nerves, you are pleased to have this interview opportunity. A firm handshake will convey energy; an accompanying smile and good eye contact will help the recruiter imagine how you might interact with a new patient or visiting relative. Interviewers should be sensitive to and have to take into account any nuances that determine how people behave socially. For example, cultural awareness around religious dress codes, the use of touch (i.e. in the form of a handshake), the level and consistency of eye contact and any disabilities (cognitive or physical such as visual or hearing impairment). If you have special requirements, then it is important to notify recruiters in advance so that they can accommodate your needs. This is a statutory requirement and should not adversely affect the outcome of any decision they make with respect to your employability.

It is important to retain poise and take time to comfortably organise oneself in the interview room. The layout may not be as you imagined; some interviews will use a very formal arrangement whereby a desk or table separates parties, whilst others adopt informality in the seating arrangement. Wherever possible the interviewee should strive for an open, engaged position facing the interviewers. Pay particular attention to the way in which you naturally sit and alter it where necessary so that you are upright with legs together/crossed, the shoulders and arms are relaxed and you lean slightly forward.

Maintaining an alertness and interest when questioned is also essential; mishearing a question is an easy mistake when under pressure. The pace of the interview can be controlled by both the interviewer and interviewee. The latter can ask for questions to be repeated or rephrased if the meaning is unclear. Another tactic is to ask for a moment to think through your answer before delivering it or excuse yourself to take a sip of water. There should always be water available; if not ask for a glass just in case your mouth dries up.

In summary, recruiters are looking for key qualities in your answers. A good answer will contain many, if not all, of the following 10 characteristics summarised in Box 5.3.

---

**BOX 5.3 10 qualities in a good response**

1. Well-thought through.
2. Succinct and to the point.
3. Supported by appropriate and clear examples from your own practice.
4. Talk about your *"accountability"* (NMC 2012c, 2015a).
5. Show some originality and fresh thinking in any examples you use to illustrate points. A conservative answer about infection control measures may refer solely to hand washing; a comprehensive answer which explore other measures including patient/visitor education around hand hygiene that shows depth.
6. Refer to the evidence-base underpinning your practice and make direct reference to key papers.
7. Acknowledge relevant policies, contemporary practice and professional issues.
8. Present your weaknesses in a professional and organised way and turn them into strengths.
9. Avoid apologies and repeated phrases like "You know."
10. Can only be given if you understand the question so; if you do not, ask for it to be repeated.

---

## WHAT NOT TO DO OR SAY AT INTERVIEW

You may well be encouraged by clinical staff (colleagues or friends) to apply for a job on a particular ward/area. A positive comment like "We'd love to have you here as a newly qualified" undoubtedly increases your confidence but needs to be understood within the context of employment law. Internal candidates can be seconded into roles, but fundamentally, all candidates, irrespective of background, have to apply through the correct process and be shortlisted for interview. Applications for NHS Jobs are anonymised so those shortlisting cannot be influenced by pre-existing knowledge of candidates; however, this may not apply for other employers. Assuming, on the basis of false reassurance, that you have got a job before the interview is very dangerous. Other hidden dangers may include those outlined in Figure 5.1:

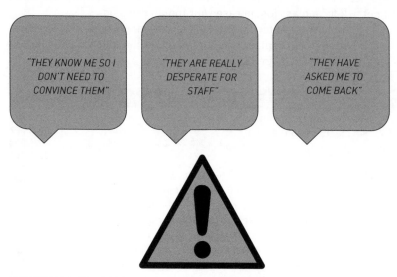

**FIGURE 5.1** The hidden dangers of assuming you've got it in the bag before the interview!

Other issues arising from a lack of self-awareness might include inappropriate attire and body language, unconscious gestures such as picking, scratching, continuously tugging at one's hair, slouching or giving limited eye contact. Are you someone who repeatedly says "You know", or "Um" when under pressure?

The use of video in mock interviews helps people see how they present and understand the negative impact and irritation that these individual nuances generate. It is best to ask your mentor for feedback but in their absence, if you can trust your family or friends to be honest and they can trust you to take it as constructive criticism, ask them to identify your two most enduring and two most irritating habits. What do they say they like or dislike about you as a person? It is not uncommon for interviewers to ask candidates "How would your friends describe you?" The outsider's view will help you prepare for this.

Inadequate preparation may manifest in the candidate who waffles their way through questions and demonstrates a very superficial level of under-standing. Remember you need to think about the purpose of a question.

Former students have relayed tales of being thrown by more obscure questions including "If you were an animal what would you be and why?" Not expecting this, one student was torn between a dolphin (because they are friendly and intelligent) and a pig. Not wishing to appear indecisive she said, "A pig, because everyone thinks that they are stupid and smell but they are actually highly intelligent, clean animals!" Whilst she felt the panel seemed impressed by this question and subsequently offered her a job, the student declined. She accepted an offer from a hospital who did not use such "bizarre" questions at interview and appeared more interested in knowing more about her as a real person and her training.

On a serious note, certain discriminatory questions are unacceptable, potentially unlawful and therefore cannot be asked by interviewers. These relate to the key areas and laws in Chapter 4, section "Applications, Interview Conduct and The Law". Applicants who declare a disability should not expect to be treated any differently from other applicants. If you are asked an inappropriate or illegal question, you must maintain professionalism. Likewise candidates are strongly discouraged from initiating discussions around controversial topics such as religion, gender relations or politics. The use of slang, derogatory terms or swearing will also undermine efforts. One employer remembers well the unsuccessful candidate who, when asked "How do you manage a stressful situation at work?" replied "I go into the locker room, bang on the lockers and shout ****, ****, ****!" and left the panel speechless.

Care is also required when referring to past employers including disputes, redundancies and unfair dismissal. For more specific information on equality and diversity visit the Target Jobs website.

It is only natural to try to gauge, by way of non-verbal and verbal cues, the interviewers' response to your answers. If they feel that your answer is incomplete, you may be offered the opportunity to add to the detail; however, this may not always happen. If you sense you have missed the point or suddenly realise that you forgot to include an essential piece of information, then you can ask to elaborate further. But again, make sure that this does not turn into waffle.

If you truly do not know the answer, then honesty is by far the best response. Imagine you are in practice, you are asked a question about medication and you do not know the answer. The recruiter is looking for assurance that you are fundamentally a safe practitioner and to this end, if you can demonstrate how and where you might find an answer, this will at least show initiative and a recognition about the limits of your competence and your accountability (NMC 2012c, 2015a).

## CLOSING THE INTERVIEW

In drawing the interview to a close, it is usual for the panel to offer you the chance to pose questions to them. A well-prepared candidate will have a list of six to eight questions based on some of the common issues in Table 5.2. Tick ones you would want answered in an interview.

| TABLE 5.2 Common issues that candidates want answered at interview | |
| --- | --- |
| **Issues** | **Tick** |
| Shift patterns | |
| Start dates for new appointees | |
| Induction procedures | |
| Preceptorship, clinical supervision and performance review | |
| Opportunities for further study and qualifications, i.e. mentorship, ILS and ALS, Learning Beyond Registration (LBR) courses | |
| Rotational post | |
| Part-time hours, flexible hours for carers, bank work and annual leave | |
| Reasonable adjustments for specific needs i.e. dyslexia, dyspraxia, a health-related issue i.e. latex allergy, diabetes or known disability | |
| Declaration of criminal record; the pre-employment DBS check will reveal any offences and may include police warnings | |
| Notification of outcome of interview | |
| Post-interview feedback and counselling | |

During the interview many of these may be addressed; however, this is another opportunity for you to demonstrate preparedness and show insight. For example, you might make reference to proposed developments within the trust strategic plan and reasonably ask how this will affect the service and what future opportunities this might open up for you. Other avenues to explore may relate to support for further study such as a degree or Master's qualification, thereby demonstrating your keenness to engage in CPD. The more obvious "When will you notify me of your decision?" and "Will you provide me with post-interview feedback, and if so how?" are ones best left to the end. If you need to ask about adjustments for dyslexia or a long-term condition then think carefully and seek advice on how to frame the question. Activity 5.3 helps you to prepare a list in advance.

## ACTIVITY 5.3

**Compiling a list of questions to ask at interview**
1. What do you need to know from the recruiter?
2. Look at the list of issues in the Table 5.2 that you have ticked.
3. Use these ticked issues to write a list of six to eight questions you will take to interview.
4. Put them in list of priority.
5. Ask a critical friend for their thoughts on the appropriateness and wording.
6. Adjust accordingly.
7. Practice these aloud.

It is common courtesy and good practice to thank the interview panel for this experience and to shake hands before leaving the room. Remain composed and professional until you are out of sight!

## LOOK AFTER NUMBER ONE!

You have worked hard to get to this point, but do not let your guard down. Often there will be students you know who are going for the same job. Read Alice's story – this is about making sure you protect your own interests and do not inadvertently give someone else an unfair advantage. Imagine how you might feel. As tempting as it is to ask for an insight into the questions, the student should not have done so (Box 5.4).

### BOX 5.4 Letting the cat out of the bag!

"There were 3 days of interviews and mine was on the Monday. Paul, our tutor, had told us not to speak to other students who had interviews before us, so I was furious when a very good friend in my tutor group texted me to say she was really nervous about her interview on Thursday and could I text her all the questions and how I answered please! Aargh! I could not believe that a close friend of mine would even ask me this when we were all going for the same jobs. I did not answer her text but found out that another close friend did. I spoke to the friend that told her all the questions and said, 'Why did you do that? How will you feel if she gets a job and we don't?' The irony of the story is, the person who divulged all the questions and answers to the other student did not get offered a position and had to re-apply, which I am sure was extremely stressful. I am happy to say she was offered a position at her second round of interviews, but what a stupid thing to do."

## HOW TO MANAGE THE OUTCOME

## MANAGING SUCCESS

Congratulations! You have been offered a job! And of course you feel on top of the world. Just one tip here – a successful interviewee needs to understand why they have been selected so that they can build on positive elements of their performance in subsequent interviews. You are just as entitled to ask for feedback from the recruiter as those who were not successful.

Some applicants may have a number of interviews, receive more than one offer and thereby be faced with making a choice between offers. Situations can be complex and difficult particularly if the applicant's first choice is not the first offer. In Boxes 5.5 and 5.6 there are several dilemmas and corresponding guidance from an experienced recruiter. You never know when you may need to go back to the person or organisation whose job offer you have turned down so these situations need to be carefully thought through. The recruitment process is a costly one and employers need to know if and why you have changed your mind.

### BOX 5.5 Jake's dilemma

Jake has put in several applications for jobs with different organisations. He is thrilled to get invited to two interviews. The interviews are a week apart and importantly the interview for the job he really wants is the second interview, not the first. He does not know whether he should attend both but thinks it would be good experience. He is worried he will get a job offer after the first interview and before he attends the second interview. How should he handle this situation? Can he ask for time to consider the offer?

Our recruiter says, "This is very good news to be invited to two interviews, and the applicant should be praised for his application as he has been shortlisted twice. Jake should attend both interviews, and if offered the first job, ask if he can have some time to think about the offer. The recruiter often agrees that a 7-day limit will be applied to the offer, and the candidate must contact the recruiter once his decision has been made."

### BOX 5.6 Managing multiple job offers: Millie's dilemma

In April Millie was offered an NQN post with a local trust and she has accepted this offer. The trust has confirmed this in writing and she has returned a signed contract. She has not been told exactly which area/department she will be working in but knows that she has a job awaiting her when she qualifies. However, two months later Millie saw an advert for her "dream job", a Band 5 in a specialist unit and applied on spec. She was shortlisted and interviewed and the manager has phoned to offer her the job. She does not want to lose this "amazing" opportunity but has already accepted a job elsewhere. How should she manage this situation?

Our recruiter advises that "Millie needs to contact the original recruiter, preferably by phone and confirm she is withdrawing from this position as soon as possible."

## MANAGING REJECTION

This is a longer section for good reason. In the unfortunate event that you did not succeed, and this will happen to everyone at some point in their careers, an insight into where you went amiss is essential. The word "success" derives from the Latin "succedere", "to come after" and Bloch (2013) reminds us that success often follows failure. Sometimes recruiters have to make choices between candidates of seemingly similar standard, so the reasons for being turned down may relate to finer detail rather than significant deficits. In some senses it is good to know that you were a clear favourite and a good runner-up.

At a time when you are feeling rejected and potentially quite emotionally fragile, approaching recruiters for feedback needs courage and careful judgement. Rejection is without doubt painful and bound to dent confidence. The adage "Never send a message in anger" or indeed when upset applies to all correspondence from phone calls, texts and emails to more formal letters.

The person delivering this news to you will anticipate a disappointed and possibly distressed response; if you do not feel able to have a meaningful conversation ask them if you can call back giving yourself time to take on board the decision and compose yourself. Better still, sleep on your frustrations and review it in the clear light of day when you have had time to reflect on how and why you feel like you do. In Box 5.7 Steve talks about his experience of handling failure.

---

**BOX 5.7 Steve's experience**

"I did fail at the first hurdle and did not get the first job I got interviewed for. I received useful feedback and used it to secure a job in the trust that I wanted.

What were the reasons for the failed first attempt? Nerves mostly! And I realise that you can't teach to prevent this, but because I was afraid of babbling and waffling I did not say enough. Tell future students, 'Do not assume that 3 years of learning disabilities experience speaks for itself.' You have to tell interviewers what you can offer to a role and incorporate all the professional topics covered within the course. Also I would say to those of a similar nature to me not to stop answering the question until the interviewer gives you a good indication that they have heard enough and enough 'boxes have been ticked'.

---

Accepting responsibility for your role in the interview and any perceived inadequacies is important; it is not good to start blaming the recruiter for not having seen your potential and in effect closing 'future' doors with remarks that may offend. Always remind yourself that every conversation should project professionalism and be aware that statements you make may be open to interpretation.

If you wish to reply to a letter of rejection, draft it out and again leave it for 24 hours. When you revisit it you may feel rather different and in a better position emotionally to write a more balanced response. Always start by thanking the recruiter for advising you of their decision and then express in measured terms your disappointment before asking for feedback so that you can learn from this drawback. Ask a critical friend for their opinion before you send it.

Furthermore, see this as a good opportunity to show the recruiter your receptiveness to constructive comment, a willingness to work on elements of your performance that would better illustrate your strengths and a time to discuss options. Look at the questions in Box 5.8 which you can use to clarify points and obtain the detail you need.

---

**BOX 5.8 What questions you should ask when you do not get a job offer**

- Where did I do well?
- What let me down?
- What attributes are you specifically looking for in prospective candidates?
- How might I improve my CV? My application? My interview performance?
- Do I need more experience? If so, what do you suggest?
- What other options are there within your organisation for someone in my position?

---

A large organisation like an NHS trust or independent sector providers (such as Partnerships in Care, Care UK or Virgin Care) comprise a network of people who communicate across invisible divides; support services such as HR often serve whole organisations so information is centrally held. Candidates who make a name for themselves for the wrong reasons will be remembered. Also clinical staff network both inside and outside of organisations. References will be followed up and if there are uncertainties a recruiter can ask for an additional reference before employing someone.

In summary, if you fall into a cycle of rejection after rejection then get advice. Box 5.9 contains a real student story about lessons learnt and a narrow escape.

---

**BOX 5.9 Jane's experience**

"As a mature student I have had many interviews for many different jobs in my time. However, applying for nursing roles is quite different. My first application did not result in an interview and although disappointed I did follow the advice and rang to enquire why not. On doing this I did receive some good advice that the particular area was looking for someone who REALLY wanted the job. Although I had researched the trust, I had not specified enough why I wanted to work on a particular ward.

Since then, prior to applying for any post, I have rung and requested to visit and then requested the person's permission to use their name in my application. I haven't had to visit many places as since then I have been successful in my next two applications and interviews (both resulted in job offers) and still have another interview invitation to consider! So I guess I can't stress enough how important it is to actually visit the place when applying for jobs. I did take time also to prepare for the interviews. I did visit one area and was able to make the decision that I really didn't want to work there. It just wasn't right for me and whilst any interview process is valuable experience I knew I would not be able to 'give my all' in an interview."

On rare occasions students can be offered a second chance if an interviewer feels that the first interview was adversely affected by nerves and they need the reassurance of a further interview to convince them that the candidate is indeed suitable. Rehearsing technique and example questions are vital in order to exploit this unusual opportunity. This has happened once in my experience as an academic tutor, proving that managing defeat and putting yourself back in front of the same panel can lead to a happy ending.

## SUMMARY

Interview skills can be rehearsed and questions predicted so unless it is an "on the spot" interview you cannot plan for, every opportunity should be taken to work on your performance. In the event of an offer, celebrate; in the event of rejection, reflect and take a proactive stance to do better next time.

# 6

# Employment Beyond First Post

## KEY WORDS

Transition; preceptorship; appraisals and progression; serendipity; CPD options; registration; NMC revalidation; portfolio; templates; modules; ECTS; Masters; clinical doctorate; PhD research doctorate; international students; clinical academic careers; specialist community public health nursing (SCPHN); networking; working abroad; humanitarian agencies; volunteering; nursing boards; CareerEDGE model; reflection and evaluation

As an NQN/NQM in employment you should now have greater stability in your life and some elements of your development mapped out. Cast your eye back to your original career plan. Are you in the type of role you set out to acquire when you started thinking about your first NQN/NQM post? What is your next step and how does this fit with your 3- or 5-year plan? This final chapter looks at AfC, continuing professional development and study options as well as ways to network.

## WHAT'S NEXT?

You are in your first post and an accountable professional. It probably feels like a "sink or swim" moment, but remember you have amazing resilience (as demonstrated by completing a 2, 3- or 4-year programme) and preceptorship as your "life raft" to ensure a safe transition. The period of preceptorship usually lasts about 12 months. The preceptee (NQN/NQM) will have structured support and guidance from a preceptor who is a more senior practitioner (DH 2009). In addition to attending study days for newly qualified staff, the employer may ask you to complete a personal portfolio and medications workbook. This is a time of consolidation and helps ease transition into professional practice by developing the preceptee's confidence and competence. In Box 6.1 Jess reflects back on her first 6 months since qualification.

### BOX 6.1 Reflections from an NQN – Jess's narrative

**What were the first 6 months like?**

My first 6 months after qualifying have been interesting. It has been a whirlwind experience. I had to learn so much again and it was like starting from day one of my training. For the first month especially I felt completely new; I was learning a whole new job. It really knocked my confidence. I went from an outgoing confident third-year student ready to qualify and take on the world, to a quiet, frightened newly qualified nurse.

I have had some real low points, especially at the beginning, doubting myself, unsure if I'd made the right choice. Some days on the ward were really busy, understaffed, ten discharges and endless bed moves. I'd get in the car and cry, I felt like I hadn't been a nurse and I wasn't able to give any of my patients any kind of care. Jobs were left undone and patients left unsatisfied, but I know I did everything I could and it still wasn't good enough. But it has only got better and better as the weeks went by, my confidence came back with the knowledge and experience I was gaining every day and I feel completely different now as to 6 months ago.

### What has preceptorship been like?

Preceptorship at my trust has been amazing; the education team are so supportive and inspiring. We had a total of six study days as an introduction to the unit, which were full of so much relevant and interesting information and at the end we (as a group of NQNs) had to do a presentation of something we had learnt over our preceptorship. I was given a mentor on the ward, who was incredibly supportive. We get together when we can, usually on night shifts, and go through my competencies and any queries I have. I have been able to talk to her and ward sisters about all of my struggles and worries.

### Have you got any advice for NQNs about making the most out of opportunity?

It's hard to be able to make time as an NQN but any opportunity to further your learning I'd highly recommend. Anything to make your patient's experience better can only be a good thing, right? As a student nurse I had a placement on a coronary care unit and loved it. I thought, this is where I want to work. Unfortunately there were no jobs there when I qualified, so I was offered a job on a cardiac ward which I was delighted about. I still knew a few members of staff down in the coronary care unit (CCU) and they remembered me as a student and when a job vacancy came up they approached me for the job. I was flattered and so happy. So 6 months after qualifying I am now working in my dream job. Initially I did feel sad I didn't get CCU as my first post but actually the opportunity to work on the ward first has made me a better nurse I feel. I am able to use the variety of experience and knowledge I've learnt and take it to a new environment.

### What is your overall plan and destination?

Eventually I'd like to specialise within a cardiac setting. I don't see myself as a ward manager personally. I enjoy patient care and the reward it brings with it too much. There are a team of nurses who work alongside the nurses in CCU called acute coronary syndrome (ACS) nurses, and that's where I'd eventually like to be.

Ideally there will be a healthy mix of stress and reward as you adjust to new role expectations, a change in support structures and the chance to explore the possibilities that come with the success of having qualified. There is increasing focus on how professional education programmes can facilitate transition, particularly in relation to identifying which elements of induction might reasonably be brought forward into the final year of programmes. The transition project (Kitson-Reynolds et al 2015), a collaboration between university and midwifery services, is one example of how associated "transition" activities and a passport system in the last year of a midwifery programme have helped students to consolidate and begin the necessary adjustments to the changing responsibilities associated with being an NQM. The evidence suggests that working earlier towards post-registration competencies helps bridge the gap and smooths the passage into the first post induction and preceptorship year.

And not surprisingly, as with any major life event, there are the numerous "survival guides". For new professionals these include the Newly Qualified Nurse's Handbook (Siviter 2008), the Nursing Survival guide series (Churchill-Livingstone publishers) and the Midwifery Survival Guide (Williams 2011). One advantage of the NHS recruitment cycle is that there are likely to be a number of people in the "same boat" as you, all starting their first posts as NQN/NQMs on the same day, so there is safety in numbers. Irrespective of whether or not you experience a smooth transition, it is worth reading one or two of these; amongst your peers there may be those who find it really tough at times and need the support of others who understand what they are going through.

Notwithstanding an element of serendipity (and you need to be ready with your CV to respond accordingly) some people have a very clear path mapped out with specific short- and long-term goals ultimately leading to a specialist role or independent practice. Others are worried more about surviving the transition and cannot think much beyond preceptorship. Ambition is good; however, there will be some key requirements for progression and promotion. Add to this the need to meet the statutory requirements for remaining on the professional register which were outlined earlier in Chapter 3, section "The Purpose of a CV".

## APPRAISALS AND PROGRESSION

Your induction and preceptorship programmes will have familiarised you with key organisational policies and procedures. Thereafter, as a professional you have responsibility for attending maintenance activities like updates (infection control, basic life support, moving and handling) and keeping a record of these. In addition there will be other continuing professional development (CPD) opportunities that will be important in order to achieve the prerequisites for moving through AfC pay band's incremental points at gateways within Band 5 and onto Band 6. You should have clear objectives linked to the Knowledge and Skills Framework (KSF) competencies and your performance against Band 5 role descriptors should be evaluated at your first and subsequent appraisals with your manager. In order to understand requirements of Band 6 practice you will need to examine a profile. You can either download a closest match Band 6 post from NHS Jobs or the agreed national profile (NHS Staff Council 2014a). These are discipline-specific and can be accessed via the links in Table 6.1.

**TABLE 6.1** Links to national profiles

| National Profile | Link |
|---|---|
| • Nursing<br>• Acute<br>• Neonatal<br>• Community<br>• Schools<br>• GP nursing<br>• Learning disability<br>• Mental health | www.nhsemployers.org/PayAndContracts/<br>AgendaForChange/NationalJobProfiles/<br>Documents/Combined |
| Midwifery | www.nhsemployers.org/PayAndContracts/<br>AgendaForChange/NationalJobProfiles/<br>Documents/Midwifery.pdf |
| Health visitors | www.nhsemployers.org/PayAndContracts/<br>AgendaForChange/NationalJobProfiles/<br>Documents/Health_Visitors.pdf |
| Theatre nursing | www.nhsemployers.org/PayAndContracts/<br>AgendaForChange/NationalJobProfiles/<br>Documents/Theatre_Nurses.pdf |

NHS Staff Council (2010) guidance states that all NHS staff should meet with their line manager for an annual performance appraisal and development review (PADR). This is not an isolated event; it forms part of the relationship between an employee and their manager. Managers can use their discretion to meet more frequently with a member of staff if needed.

The PADR process has two core parts (NHS Staff Council, 2010, p. 4):

- Performance appraisal is the process of agreeing personal objectives and how their achievement can be measured and then assessing how staff perform against them in the context of the organisation's goals and values.
- Personal development planning and review (PDP/R) is the process of defining the types and levels of skills, knowledge and behaviour that staff require in carrying out their work, assessing their current skill levels against these requirements and then putting development plans in place to close any gaps or shortfalls.

In readiness for these meetings employees can go to the NHS Employers website or refer to the RCN booklets (2006, 2007, 2009) where there is a wealth of information including preparing for appraisal, a simplified KSF, appraisal tools and tips for completion. As a student you will have been used to interviews as part of the assessment in practice process; this is similar and reliant on evidence of achievement. In preparation for NQN/NQM interviews you should already have a CPD portfolio (refer to section "How to Create a Portfolio for Interviews and CPD" in Chapter 3), fronted by an up-to-date CV.

Your employer will expect you to be proactive so you will need to reflect on your progress to date and give thought to what your needs are alongside the needs of the organisation and have an outline personal development plan (PDP). Have a look at the options listed in Activity 6.1 and tick those you would like to undertake or investigate further. Timescales need accounting for and of course funding may be a key

**ACTIVITY 6.1**

Options for CPD

| Opportunities | Proposed timescale | Employer-funded | Self-funded |
|---|---|---|---|
| Publish article based on dissertation studies | | | |
| Complete a recognised mentor-ship course | | | |
| Leadership skills | | | |

| | | | |
|---|---|---|---|
| Intravenous drugs | | | |
| Venepuncture and cannulation | | | |
| History taking and physical assessment | | | |
| Non-medical prescribing | | | |
| Conference attendance (local, regional, national or international) | | | |
| Join special interest group (RCN; RCM) | | | |
| Submit poster for conference (local, regional, national or international) | | | |
| Rotation within current area | | | |
| Practice visits outside of current area | | | |
| Secondment to another depart- ment (i.e. clinical or project work) | | | |
| Grants or sponsorship to help fund studies | | | |
| Degree or Master's-level modules related to current specialism | | | |
| Degree or Master's qualification (broader) | | | |
| Specialist Community Public Health Nursing (SCPHN) | | | |
| Clinical Academic Careers (including clinical doctorate or PhD) | | | |
| Voluntary work abroad (episodic) | | | |
| Work abroad | | | |
| Internship | | | |

determinant so also indicate whether or not this will be employer- or self-funded. Now you can start looking at in-house provision, your local higher education institute (HEI) provider prospectus or wider afield. It might be worth talking with more senior staff or university alumni about their career trajectories.

## CONTINUING PROFESSIONAL DEVELOPMENT

Continuing professional development (CPD), also referred to as continuing professional education (CPE), is "fundamental to the development of all health and social care practitioners, and is the mechanism through which high quality patient and client care is identified, maintained and developed" (RCN 2007b, p. 2). It is a means by which you will maintain the knowledge and skills essential to professional practice. Your obligations, as set out by the NMC (2015a, b), were previously outlined in Chapter 3, section "The Purpose of a CV". The NMC (2015b, p. 10) states that you must undertake 40 hours of CPD in the 3 years leading up to the renewal of your registration. Participatory learning must account for half (20) of these 40 hours. From day one of your first NQN/NQM post, it is important to start recording your CPD activities in a designated CPD portfolio alongside a current CV, study day programmes and certificates of attendance, neatly held within plastic folders. The CPD must be accurately recorded on the five templates that the NMC (2015c) provides. These are:

1. Practice record log
2. Continuing professional development (CPD) record log
3. Reflective accounts record log comprising five detailed reflections
4. Professional development discussion form
5. Confirmation from a third-party form

The "means" by which this development takes place is not stipulated. CPD can take a variety of different formats from attending taught modules, conference attendance, single study days or workshops, work-based learning (WBL), accredited online study or self-directed uncredited activity or visits to other departments or service providers. The type of experience should be negotiated with your manager. Table 6.2 is a checklist for completing your portfolio (NMC 2015b) to ensure that you have all the relevant information. Remember that the NMC (2015b) retains the right to audit every professional's CPD record.

| TABLE 6.2 Checklist for completing your portfolio | |
| --- | --- |
| **Requirements** | **Supporting evidence to include** |
| **Practice hours** | Maintain a record of practice hours you have completed, including:<br>• Dates of practice<br>• The number of hours you undertook<br>• Name, address and postcode of the organisation<br>• Scope of practice<br>• Work setting<br>• A description of the work you undertook<br>• Evidence of those practice hours (such as timesheets, role profiles or job specifications). |
| **Continuing professional development** | Maintain accurate and verifiable records of your CPD activities including:<br>• The CPD method<br>• A brief description of the topic and how it relates to your practice<br>• Dates the CPD activity was undertaken<br>• The number of hours and participatory hours<br>• Identification of the part of the Code most relevant to the CPD<br>• Evidence of the CPD activity (Annex 2 in the guidance provides examples of the kind of evidence you can record in your portfolio). |
| **Practice-related feedback** | Notes of the content of the feedback and how you used it to improve your practice. This will be helpful for you to use when you are preparing your reflective accounts. |
| **Reflection and discussion** | Five reflective accounts that explain what you learnt from the CPD activity or feedback, how you changed or improved your work as a result and how it is relevant to the Code.<br><br>A reflection and discussion form which includes the name and NMC PIN of the registrant that you had the discussion with as well as the date you had the discussion. |
| **Health and character** | These declarations will be made as part of your online revalidation application. You do not need to keep anything in your portfolio as part of this requirement. |

| TABLE 6.2 *continued* | |
| --- | --- |
| **Requirements** | **Supporting evidence to include** |
| **Professional indemnity arrangement** | Whether your indemnity arrangement is through your employer, a membership with a professional body or through a private insurance arrangement. |
| | If your indemnity arrangement is provided by membership with a professional body or a private insurance arrangement, you will need to record the name of the professional body or provider. |
| | Evidence to demonstrate that you have an appropriate arrangement in place. |
| **Third-party confirmation** | A signed confirmation form. |

Source: NMC 2015b, pp. 31–32.

Taking an accredited module gives you the ideal chance to partici-pate in rigorous academic study. To apply for a stand-alone module or short course you should first discuss your interest with your manager as employer support, by way of days allocated for attendance and finan-cial funding, may be available. In addition, you may be very lucky and secure extra ring-fenced time for associated independent study, but more often than not employees have to learn how best to manage study alongside their usual work commitments.

Some HEI modules such as mentorship, history taking and physical assessment, prescribing and leadership will have been commissioned by trusts and other organisations. This means that there will be a num-ber of allocated places, based on priority workplace needs as identified by the employer. As a result, the selection you are offered could be restricted; if you wish to do a module that is not a prerequisite for your role or essential for your future development, you will need to compile a robust case to support an application or consider self-funding.

Assessed modules, as opposed to attendance only, will have academic credit attached. Each one is worth 5–20 credits under the European Credit Transfer System (ECTS). The same system operates with undergraduate degrees so you should be familiar with this. The employer might stipulate that undertaking the assessed component of a module is a requirement; for example, with mentorship where mentors have to have completed and passed a recognised mentorship course in order to undertake the role of a mentor. However, if continuing in formal study is not for you at this moment in time, modules, study days and summer schools can often be taken without the assessment, solely for the purposes of CPD.

## BOX 6.4 The clinical academic career: Mat's journey

I would argue that my first exposure to a clinical academic career was during my 3-year undergraduate training as a student nurse. During the training I grew to like how the course was divided into two distinct blocks of clinical placements and academic instruction. I particularly liked how clinical placements broke the monotony of academic periods and vice versa. It is no wonder that as the course was coming to an end, I was conflicted as to which career pathway to follow as I presumed that pursuing a clinical career pathway meant sacrificing the academic career pathway and vice versa. I was therefore delighted when my local university offered me the opportunity to become a clinical academic. I was offered the opportunity to undertake PhD studies linked to any clinical area of my choice. The university entered into an agreement with me whereby they would let me choose the clinical area that I wanted to work in, and in turn they would draft a PhD project based on that clinical area. True to the agreement, I chose to work in the acute medical unit of a local hospital and the university drafted a research proposal related to the unit after consulting with the unit's matron. Now I work two clinical days a week as a nurse in the acute medical unit and three academic days a week as a PhD student.

My advice to students who are contemplating pursuing a clinical academic career pathway similar to mine would be as follows: "Please do not allow yourself to be naive about the following important truths. Firstly, you will be undertaking a significant academic leap from undergraduate (or postgraduate diploma) studies into PhD studies, and secondly, you will be undertaking a significant professional leap from student nurse (without official banding) to newly qualified nurse (with a Band 5 banding that carries enormous responsibility)."

Both leaps are equally exciting and terrifying and will require you to have the humility to accept the fact that you need substantial academic and clinical support. They will also require you to have a stubborn resilience firmly grounded in your desire to want to get that PhD and be the best hands on nurse that you can be. My high and low moments so far as a clinical academic have revolved around humility and resilience. Humility helps me to acknowledge my weaknesses; resilience helps me to address them without feeling defeated by them. For example, I acknowledge that undertaking PhD studies does not equate to clinical skills; however, instead of accepting the popular notion that my clinical skills will never be as good as those of my clinical peers, I seek appropriate support and opportunities to attain and maintain the same clinical skills as my peers. In fact, only recently I managed to secure a post as a clinical practice educator who facilitates the development of newly qualified nurses – testimony to the fact that I am considered to be a highly skilled and competent clinician.

As for the future, I hope to complete my PhD studies and possibly enrol into the NIHR/HEE CAT Clinical Lectureship Scheme. More importantly, however, I hope that YOU will actively consider pursuing a clinical academic career as it is quite rewarding.

You may also like to refer to my online profile using the link below:

www.uhs.nhs.uk/Research/Research-for-nurses-midwives-andAHPs/Examples-and-experiences/Improving-DV-management-in-acute-care.aspx

## SPECIALIST COMMUNITY PUBLIC HEALTH NURSING (SCPHN)

The government (DH 2011) is investing resources in order to train 4200 more registered health visitors (HV) by 2015. As a result, there are numerous SCPHN courses available around the UK. The NMC (2011b) has stated there is no minimum period of post-registration experience required to undertake HV training. If you are a registered nurse or midwife you can move your career forward with this community nursing qualification, which will improve leadership and management skills. As a result you are eligible for employment as a health visitor, school nurse, occupational health nurse or sexual health practitioner. This SCPHN qualification is recorded on Part 3 of the NMC Register. In Box 6.5 Sonia outlines her route to this qualification.

### BOX 6.5 SCPHN: Sonia's route to qualification

I have just qualified as a midwife on the 3-year BMid (Hons). Midway through my final year I applied to the local NHS Trust for the position of student specialist community public health nurse (health visitor) and was invited to attend an interview. I was successful! This meant that I knew that when I qualified I would be employed by the trust and supported to study a postgraduate diploma at the university with a clinical placement in the local area.

At the start of the interview introductions were made with the interview panel and other interviewees and relevant paperwork collected. Our first task was a group activity. We were given a subject

Any overseas travel where you wish to work in a professional capacity needs careful planning; this may include you undertaking additional study. The process can be extremely lengthy and arduous so you need to be extremely patient and be realistic with timescales. The RCN website provides factsheets on the popular destinations and links to RCN members/contacts based overseas. These are three key references:

- www.rcn.org.uk/nursing/working_overseas
- www.rcn.org.uk/__data/assets/pdf_file/0008/590732/General-information-on-working-abroad-v4.pdf
- www.rcn.org.uk/__data/assets/pdf_file/0007/347920/Working_with_humanitarian_organisations.2010.pdf

Volunteering with a charitable organisation such as Raleigh can be life-enhancing. In Box 6.6 Sarah talks about how she successfully combines her NHS work with ad hoc volunteering in India and Uganda, and with the Red Cross in Sierra Leone. A post-qualifying course in Tropical medicine prepared her for tough times with little or no resources except her clinical skills to fall back on.

---

### BOX 6.6 Sarah's reflections on combining work and volunteering

Before commencing my nurse training I was actively involved volunteering with organisations such as Girl Guiding UK, Millennium Volunteers and the Prince's Trust. I developed a love for volunteering; being able to give back to the community is extremely rewarding but I have also developed a variety of skills and had lots of fun along the way.

These initial volunteering experiences inspired me to take a gap year before university in Uganda (2006). For several months I volunteered in a small school for orphans, with the majority of children in some way affected by prevalent diseases such as HIV/AIDS, tuberculosis and malaria. Health awareness was minimal and most children were also affected by problems such as malnutrition and sanitation-related problems such as waterborne diseases and parasitic infections. It was at this point I realised that I had developed an interest in healthcare and what I could do, especially in developing countries, to help others.

I was grateful to be accepted by the university in 2006 to study Adult Nursing. So I began 3 years of lectures and on-the-job training. In my final year, I was able to undertake my professional development experience in Mukono Clinic, in Uganda. This time around, having gained several years' experience working in clinical settings, I was able to contribute far more to the people and environment I worked in. I realised that my passion lay in using my skills as a nurse in disadvantaged settings abroad.

As soon as I qualified in 2009 I undertook a Postgraduate Diploma in Tropical Nursing on a part-time basis whilst also working in the Acute Medical Admissions Unit (AMU) at the General Hospital. The diploma gave me an excellent insight into the causes, prevention and treatment of major tropical diseases as well as cultural, structural and organisational aspects of working in resource-poor settings. Meanwhile, working on AMU allowed me to develop transferable skills and gain knowledge in nursing a variety of acute conditions. In 2013, I decided to seek out new opportunities and following on from some time volunteering in Uganda again, I was lucky enough to secure work with Raleigh International in south India.

Raleigh "International Citizen Service" is a development-orientated programme with an emphasis on cross-cultural learning. As a medic, another colleague and I were responsible for the health and well-being of around 140 UK and Indian volunteers, aged 18–25, as well as in-country staff. With volunteers often in remote areas I learnt to think on my feet, to trust in my judgement and to utilise all the skills I had gained since my training began. I was excited to be able to see first-hand and diagnose tropical illnesses such as Dengue Fever. I also spent time teaching Health and Hygiene, BLS and Moving and Handling to all the volunteers and team leaders. It was very rewarding seeing the teams pass this knowledge on to villagers in their project sites when giving health awareness classes and seeing the difference it made to individuals and communities.

Following the 2014 Ebola outbreak in West Africa, I started work for the British Red Cross in Sierra Leone, working alongside national nurses and international delegates. Given the severity of the disease, I undertook extensive training in Geneva before deployment. Ebola is known to be highly contagious and as such, all nursing staff need to wear full protective clothing, similar to hazmat suits, in order to remain safe when working in direct contact with patients in the high-risk zone. In Geneva we practised safely getting in and out of these suits, to maintain safety, and also studied the cultural context and history of the outbreak. Arriving in Sierra Leone, nothing could have prepared me for the devastation caused by the Ebola outbreak. Treatment centres were full to capacity and the strain on health services was apparent. As a team, we adopted basic nursing practices due to limited resources. There were no blood gas machines, complicated infusions or invasive monitoring that we come to learn about and rely on as nurses working in the UK. Instead we relied on our ability to diagnose and treat using our eyes, our ears, our skills and our knowledge. This was extremely rewarding and made me appreciate how much I have learnt over the years, from different settings and experiences. Although there were of course difficult times working in such an outbreak, there were also amazing moments, the type that remind me why I love being a nurse.

| Nursing Times | www.nursingtimes.net |
|---|---|
| Prospects | www.prospects.ac.uk<br>*(UK Official Graduate Careers Website for General Careers Information and Graduate Vacancies)* |
| Queen Alexandra's Royal Army Nursing Corps | www.army.mod.uk/medical-services/nursing.aspx |
| Royal Air Force | www.raf.mod.uk/recruitment/ |
| Royal College of Midwives | www.rcm.org.uk |
| Royal College of Nursing | www.rcn.org.uk<br>www.rcnpublishing.com/page/ns/courses-and-careers/career-advice/career-development<br>www.rcn.org.uk/development/learning/learningzone<br>www.rcni.com/portfolio<br>*(RCNi portfolio; revalidation support; CPD resources)* |
| Royal College of Nursing Immigration Advice Service | www.rcn.org.uk/support/services/immigration_advice_service |
| Royal Navy | www.royalnavy.mod.uk |
| Target Jobs | targetjobs.co.uk/careers-advice/equality-and-diversity<br>targetjobs.co.uk/careers-advice/interview-techniques<br>targetjobs.co.uk/careers-advice/psychometric-tests/275677-psychometric-tests-what-they-are-and-why-graduates-need-to-know |
| Home Office UK Border Agency (UKBA) | www.gov.uk/browse/visas-immigration |

| NURSING AND MIDWIFERY CAREERS ABROAD | |
|---|---|
| Nursing and Midwifery Board of Ireland | www.nursingboard.ie/en/homepage.aspx |
| Australian Nursing and Midwifery Accreditation Council (ANMAC) | www.anmc.org.au |
| Nursing and Midwifery Board of Australia | www.nursingmidwiferyboard.gov.au |
| Nursing Council for New Zealand | www.nursingcouncil.org.nz |

| National Council of States Boards of Nursing (NCSBN) (North America) | www.ncsbn.org/index.htm |
|---|---|
| Nurse Licensure Compact (North America) | www.ncsbn.org/nlc.htm |
| Nursys | www.nursys.com<br>*(National database for verification of nurse licensure in North America)* |
| National Nursing Assessment Service (Canada) | www.nnas.ca/about-us |
| Commission on Graduates of Foreign Nursing Schools | www.cgfns.org<br>*(Credentials evaluation service)* |
| International Council of Nurses | www.icn.ch/what-we-do/global-database/<br>www.icn.ch/what-we-do/regulation/the-role-and-identity-of-the-regulator/global-database/contact-information-sheet.html<br>*(Contact sheet for nursing organisations by country)* |
| Royal College of Nursing | www.rcn.org.uk/nursing/workingabroad |

| OTHER USEFUL RESOURCES | |
|---|---|
| British National Formulary/BNF for Children | www.medicinescomplete.com |
| NMC Standards for Medicines Management | www.nmc.org.uk/standards/additional-standards/standards-for-medicines-management/ |
| SafeMedicate | www.safeMedicate.com<br>*(E-Learning software for developing and assessing competence for safe drug calculations)* |
| The International English Language Testing System (IELTS) Exam | www.ielts.org |

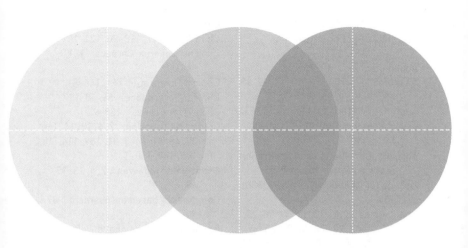

# Index